HEALING YOUR GRIEVING HEART AFTER A CANCER DIAGNOSIS

D0710836

Also by Alan Wolfelt and Kirby Duvall:

*Healing a Friend or Loved One's
Grieving Heart After a Cancer Diagnosis:
100 Practical Ideas for Providing
Compassion, Comfort, and Care*

*Healing Your Grieving Body:
100 Physical Practices for Mourners*

*Healing After Job Loss:
100 Practical Ideas*

Also by Alan Wolfelt:

*Healing Your Grieving Heart:
100 Practical Ideas*

*The Journey Through Grief:
Reflections on Healing*

*The Mourner's Book of Hope:
30 Days of Inspiration*

*Understanding Your Grief:
Ten Essential Touchstones for Finding
Hope and Healing Your Heart*

*Companion Press is dedicated to the education and
support of both the bereaved and bereavement caregivers.
We believe that those who companion the bereaved by
walking with them as they journey in grief have a
wondrous opportunity: to help others embrace and grow
through grief—and to lead fuller, more deeply-lived lives
themselves because of this important ministry.*

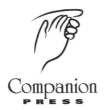

Companion
P R E S S

For a complete catalog and ordering information, write, call, or visit:

Companion Press
The Center for Loss and Life Transition
3735 Broken Bow Road
Fort Collins, CO 80526
(970) 226-6050
www.centerforloss.com

HEALING YOUR GRIEVING HEART
AFTER A CANCER DIAGNOSIS

•

100 PRACTICAL IDEAS FOR
COPING, SURVIVING, AND THRIVING

•

ALAN D. WOLFELT, PH.D.
KIRBY J. DUVALL, M.D.

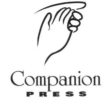

Companion
PRESS

An imprint of the Center for Loss and Life Transition
Fort Collins, Colorado

Companion Press is an imprint of the
Center for Loss and Life Transition
3735 Broken Bow Road
Fort Collins, Colorado 80526
970-226-6050

Companion Press titles may be purchased in bulk for sales promotions, premiums, or fundraisers. Please contact the publisher at the above address for more information.

Printed in the United States of America

21 20 19 18 17 16 15 14   5 4 3 2 1

ISBN: 978-1-61722-200-9

In Gratitude

To the people who have been willing to share their cancer journeys with us and inspired us to pen this resource.

CONTENTS

INTRODUCTION

Thank you for picking up this book. You probably have it in your hands because you have been diagnosed with some form of cancer. We are so sorry you had to hear these difficult words: "You have cancer."

We wish you courage, grace, comfort, and hope as you begin to explore this resource. Please view this little book as an encouraging friend who takes your hand and walks with you, by your side. As good friends do, let it fill you with the strength and belief that you cannot only survive your cancer but go on to discover new meaning and purpose in your life.

My personal story

I was riding my bike in the gorgeous mountains outside of Aspen, Colorado. The day was bright and beautiful. I was enjoying spending the day with my precious daughter Megan and two of her close friends. The furthest thing from my head and heart was anything related to cancer.

Just as I was rounding a slight bend on the bike trail, my cell phone rang. Despite taking a day off for renewal, I had some instinct to answer the call. The female voice on the other end of the line did not mince words. "Is this Dr. Wolfelt?" she asked matter-of-factly. "Yes, it is," I responded. She quickly proceeded. "I'm sorry to have to tell you this on the telephone, but your biopsy results came back, and you have prostate cancer."

I could not move. I could not bring myself to utter even a word in response to her statement. Upon reflection, I don't think I wanted the word "cancer" to register with me. My initial response was anchored in a combination of shock, fear, and protest. I don't remember any words that passed between us after I heard those dreaded words, "You have cancer."

When the shock evolved to overwhelming sadness, I began to think about how I didn't want to leave my wife, Sue, and my three beloved children, Megan, Chris, and Jaimie. I said to myself, "Is this it? Am I going to die in my fifties? What if I don't survive this? I have so much to live for, more love to give, more books to write, more workshops to teach. I'm not ready to go!" This was the start of my rollercoaster ride of self-examination, personal discovery, and even some "enforced learning of life."

Oh yes, if anyone inappropriately tells you that "you will grow from this" or "It will make you a better person," remember the word "enforced." This was not for me, and will not be for you, growth you would choose. Actually, you would choose to have your health back!

Not only am I a cancer survivor, I am a grief counselor and educator. For more than thirty years, I have taught people about the need to embrace and express their grief after a significant loss so they can go on to live and love well again. This book, then, sits squarely at the intersection of two important pieces of my life. I am honored to walk beside you on your journey.

You and I are among the more than 13 million Americans alive today (and hundreds of millions more the world over) who have faced a cancer diagnosis. We have this in common, yet each of us is unique. We come to cancer with our own personal and family histories, our unique personalities, our own ways of dealing with challenges and loss. Even when we share a diagnosis or prognosis, our circumstances vary tremendously. Your cancer journey will be as unique as you are. Yet despite our differences, there is comfort in knowing that none of us walks alone.

Cancer is loss

Cancer is a significant loss. No matter your type or stage of cancer or survivorship, your life changed after your diagnosis. From the moment you first heard those three little words, you experienced losses of many kinds.

You lost your health. Even if you recovered your health in the months and years after your treatment, you know what it means to feel healthy one moment and frighteningly unhealthy the next.

You lost your sense of normalcy and safety. Your life was going along in its usual way when *wham!*—you were broadsided by cancer. Few diseases turn life so topsy-turvy for such a long period of time. And the uncertainty of your prognosis likely made you feel unsafe and anxious—for yourself as well as for those who love you and depend on you.

If your treatment was extensive or ongoing, you may have lost your ability to work, as well. You may have lost financial stability.

In the course of your treatment, perhaps you lost a body part or two, your hair, your appetite, your memory (thanks to chemo brain), and even some of your friends. Not everyone is capable of the steadfastness it takes to be a friend through the cancer journey.

So yes, in myriad ways, cancer is synonymous with loss. And when we lose things (or people) that we care about or that are important to our sense of self, we naturally grieve.

Grief is what we think and feel on the inside when we lose someone or something important. When someone we love dies, for example, we experience shock, anger, guilt, sadness, and other emotions. We think many dark and difficult thoughts. All of these thoughts and feelings go into a pot called grief.

Mourning your grief

You have grieved since your cancer diagnosis, I am sure. I know I did, and I continue to do so. Those who love us have grieved too. The purpose of this book is to help you embrace grief as normal and necessary and find ways to express it outside yourself.

Mourning is the word for grief expressed. While grief is what's bottled up inside you, mourning is the opening up, the letting out, and the sharing.

Without mourning, grief festers. Contrary to the cliché "time heals all wounds," grief does not magically dissipate through the passage of time alone. If it is not expressed fully and honestly, it tends to result in ongoing problems such as depression, intimacy troubles, chronic anxiety, substance abuse, and others.

But *with* mourning? Oh, with mourning, what rich rewards await us on the far side of grief! When genuinely expressed, grief has the potential to open us to a richer and deeper experience of life. We cancer club members sometimes roll our eyes or get annoyed at all the talk about the "gifts of cancer." But it's true. Cancer can and does bring us gifts, but only if we express our thoughts and feelings and connect with those around us.

You'll probably notice that here and there throughout this book I use the word "healing" when I'm talking about grief. Expressing your cancer grief—that is, mourning your cancer grief—is how you heal in the spiritual/emotional sense. I do not mean to be insensitive with the term "healing," however, and I understand that when you have a life-threatening illness, you may naturally be focused on healing your physical body and living a long life, cancer-free. While I do believe in the power of mind-body connection, I would never be so irresponsible as to suggest that mourning openly and fully will heal your cancer. What I do believe is that it will help you cope with your cancer and live fully and on purpose. It will help you survive and thrive—no matter how many weeks, months, or years you may yet live and breathe on this Earth.

How to use this book

I wrote this book together with my longtime friend and physician Dr. Kirby Duvall. To my passion about helping others in grief and my own cancer survivorship, he adds decades of medical experience helping patients who have cancer. While this is more of a spiritual guide to cancer than a medical one, his medical expertise informs many of the ideas you'll find here.

As promised, this book contains 100 ideas to help support you as you mourn your cancer grief. Some of the ideas will teach you about the principles of grief and mourning. One of the most important ways to help yourself is to learn about the grief experience. The remainder of the 100 ideas offer practical, here-and-now, action-oriented suggestions for embracing your grief and practicing self-compassion. Each idea is followed by a brief explanation of how and why the idea might help you.

Some of the ideas will speak to your unique experience better than others. If you come to an idea that doesn't seem to fit you, simply ignore it and turn to another page.

As you flip through these pages, you will also see that each idea includes a "Carpe Diem," which means, as fans of the movie *Dead Poets Society* will remember, "seize the day." Our hope is that you not relegate this resource to your shelves but instead keep it handy on your nightstand or desk. Pick it up often and turn to any page; the Carpe Diem suggestion might help you seize the day by giving you an exercise, action, or thought to consider today, right now, right this minute.

Please understand that nothing is this book should be construed as medical advice. If you have questions or concerns about any medical matter, you should consult your doctor or other healthcare provider. You should never delay seeking medical advice, disregard medical advice, or discontinue medical treatment because of information contained in this book.

We thank you for taking the time to read and reflect on the words that make up this book. We wish you courage, grace, and comfort on your cancer journey. Please view this little book as an encouraging companion who walks with you.

Godspeed. We hope to meet you one day.

Alan D. Wolfelt

1.

UNDERSTAND THE DIFFERENCE BETWEEN GRIEF AND MOURNING

"What happens when people open their hearts?
They get better."
— Haruki Murakami

- Grief is the constellation of internal thoughts and feelings we experience when we lose something or someone we care about. Grief is the weight in the chest, the churning in the gut, the unspeakable thoughts and feelings.

- Mourning is the outward expression of our grief. Mourning is crying, journaling, creating artwork, talking to others, telling the story, speaking the unspeakable.

- Here's a way to remember which is which: The "i" in grief stands for what I feel inside. The "u" in mourn reminds me to share my grief with you.

- Everyone grieves when they are affected by life's challenges, but if we are to heal emotionally and spiritually, we must also mourn. Over time, and with the support of others, to mourn is to heal.

- Many of the ideas in this book are intended to help you mourn the natural and necessary grief that has resulted from your cancer diagnosis and ongoing treatment.

CARPE DIEM
Ask yourself this question: Have I been mourning my cancer, or have I mostly been restricting myself to grieving?

2.

ALLOW FOR NUMBNESS

"There is a feeling of disbelief that comes over you, that takes over, and you kind of go through the motions. You do what you're supposed to do, but in fact you're not there at all."
— Frederick Barthelme

- Did you feel numb and in shock in the days and weeks right after your cancer diagnosis? I know I did and sometimes still do.

- Feelings of shock, numbness, and disbelief are nature's way of temporarily protecting us from the full force of a painful reality. Like anesthesia, these feelings help us survive the pain of our early grief. Be thankful for numbness.

- We often think, "I will wake up and this will not have happened." Early mourning can feel like being in a dream. Your emotions need time to catch up with what your mind has been told.

- Cancer typically requires many, many doctors' visits and tests and procedures. This means that at the same time you are feeling numb and not thinking well, you are being given lots of complex information and sometimes have to make difficult decisions based on your understanding of that information. Ask a friend or family member to accompany you to appointments, take notes, and help you decide.

CARPE DIEM
If you're feeling numb, cancel any optional commitments that require concentration and decision-making. Allow yourself time to regroup. Find a "safe haven" that you might be able to retreat to for a few days.

3.

TAKE AN INVENTORY

"The minute someone tells you you have cancer, it's kind of like you die. You really do die. It's like you get that you're mortal."
— Eve Ensler

- When you were diagnosed with cancer, you lost not only your health (at least somewhat and temporarily) but so much more.
- You may have lost your hold on your hopes and dreams for your future as well as your family's future.
- You may have lost your sense of security and safety—for yourself and for others who depend on you.
- If you had surgery, you lost a part of yourself.
- You may have lost closeness or intimacy with loved ones.
- You may have lost some of your physical abilities and pleasures.
- You may have lost some of your faith in God.
- You may have lost your trust in medicine or in your own body.
- You may have lost financial stability.
- You may have lost your trust in how life is supposed to work.
- It's no wonder that cancer grief can feel so heavy.

CARPE DIEM
Today, take an inventory of all you have lost as a result of your diagnosis and prognosis. Write it down and/or talk about it with someone who's a good listener and is able to be supportive to you.

4.

GIVE YOURSELF PERMISSION TO GRIEVE AND MOURN

"It is so important to talk about your cancer and the feelings you have about it."

— Mindy Sterling

- As we discussed in this book's Introduction, being diagnosed and living with cancer creates many losses. And with loss comes natural and necessary grief. Your grief is very real, and it will affect you physically, emotionally, socially, intellectually, and spiritually.

- Sometimes people with cancer set aside or discount their own grief. Sometimes they are so focused on worrying about and supporting their loved ones that they neglect themselves. Sometimes they take a look at other cancer patients around them and think, "Lots of people have it worse than I do. I have nothing to complain about." But the truth is, you are grieving inside, and rightfully so.

- If you enjoy life and if you love and are connected to others, cancer threatens all of that—in many ways. You will likely try to minimize the threat by accepting the best treatment available, but still, the threat barged into your life and will probably, at least to some extent, remain forever.

- You need and deserve the healing gifts of mourning. We invite you to use this book to acquaint yourself with a variety of ways to mourn openly and honestly.

CARPE DIEM

Today, talk to someone about your cancer journey. Tell them the medical facts if you like, but more important, tell them how those facts make you feel inside.

5.

LOVE YOURSELF

"If there is a panacea or cure-all to life, it is self-love."
— Paul Solomon

- Someone once astutely observed, "Love is the highest, purest, most precious of all spiritual things." It is easier to express love to others than it is to ourselves. Yet, by feeling your own love more surely, you can be transformed and open yourself to hope and healing.

- Loving yourself starts with accepting yourself. If you, as a living, unique human being, are unable to value who you are, who can? If part of your need to mourn is anchored in recapturing your capacity to give love out, you must start by giving love in. You need to honor yourself right now. Nobody else can do it from the inside out.

- Loving yourself means recognizing you, seeing you, and honoring you. In part, it is about celebrating yourself. It is a privilege to be you, cancer or no cancer. You have been given the opportunity to feel, to see, to live life with both its challenges and opportunities. Sometimes, in the midst of the pain of your grief, you can forget this. You may feel alone, questioning your existence, not liking who you are, and being self-disparaging. Yet, even in the face of loss, remember: It is a gift to be alive, and just being born into the world is a compliment. Being able to give and receive love and then mourn your life losses is part of the beauty of being alive. If you forget to affirm the truth that "blessed are those who mourn," you insult the consciousness that gave you life.

CARPE DIEM
Dedicate this day to loving yourself. Find a quiet place to sit in stillness. Now, remind yourself of your inner beauty and unique self. Befriend your emotional and spiritual strengths, your humor, your intelligence, your sensitivity, your wisdom, your gifts. From this conscious, loving acceptance, your capacity to eventually open yourself to loving life again—even with cancer!—can come forth.

6.

FOCUS ON FIRST THINGS FIRST

"What happens when my body breaks down happens not just to that body but also to my life, which is lived in that body. When the body breaks down, so does the life."

— Arthur Frank

- Have you ever seen the psychologist Abraham Maslow's famous "hierarchy of needs"? It's a pyramid that shows the natural and normal priority of human needs.

- The base of the pyramid is formed by our physiological needs—in other words, the needs of our bodies. If you're in the middle of 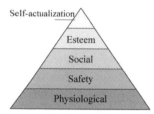 treatment right now, your body is under attack and will likely demand all your attention for a while. Get ample rest, eat as well as you can, stay hydrated, and ask for help with any pain you might be experiencing.

- Don't assume that you simply have to bear pain. If you are hurting, talk to your doctors about it. Ask to see a pain care specialist if need be. Controlling your pain as much as possible is essential to not just surviving but actually living in the weeks to come.

- Until your needs for physical comfort and safety are met, you simply can't move up the pyramid to address your social, emotional, and spiritual needs.

- Every day, focus on first things first. Take good care of yourself physically. Only if you are feeling well enough will you be able to engage with the people who care about you and with your own spirit. To focus on your own physical needs first is a strength, not a weakness.

CARPE DIEM

Ask yourself: How am I feeling physically right now, this very minute? Am I tired? Hungry? Stiff? In pain? Attend to your physical needs immediately.

7.

KEEP A JOURNAL

"From time to time, I'll look back through the personal journals I've scribbled in throughout my life, the keepers of my raw thoughts and emotions. The words poured forth after my dad died, when I went through a divorce, and after I was diagnosed with breast cancer. There are so many what-ifs scribbled on those pages."

— Hoda Kotb

- Cancer is a journey. So is grief.

- Have you ever noticed how the word "journey" and "journal" are similar? Both come from the French word *jour*, which means "day." As you journey through cancer and grief, one day a time, consider capturing your daily thoughts, feelings, and experiences in a journal.

- Even if you don't think of yourself as a writer and have never journaled before, I encourage you to give it a try now. Journaling is a form of outward expression of your interior reality. It's mourning! And as I've emphasized, mourning is how you move toward healing your grief and living and loving fully.

- Don't worry about the quality of your writing. That doesn't matter in the least. The only thing that matters is the honest expression and exploration of what you are thinking and feeling inside.

CARPE DIEM

Pick up a journal or empty notebook today and write for at least 15 minutes without stopping. See what comes out. Do it again tomorrow.

8.

UNDERSTAND THE SIX NEEDS OF MOURNING

Need #1: Acknowledge the reality of your diagnosis and prognosis

"Everything was going for me. I didn't even know the meaning of the word 'insecurity' and suddenly I am surrounded by words like 'operation,' 'cancer,' 'chemotherapy,' 'radiation.'"

— Delta Goodrem

- You have cancer. This is a difficult reality to accept. Yet gently, slowly, and patiently, you must embrace this reality, bit by bit, day by day.

- If you are in the early weeks and months of your cancer journey, you may still be struggling to accept this reality. It's common for this need of mourning to take a while. You will first acknowledge the reality of your cancer with your head. Only over time will you come to acknowledge it with your heart.

- If you are many months or years into your cancer journey, you have probably come to acknowledge this reality. You have probably learned to live in the uncertain world of probabilities and maybes.

- Growing comfortable with speaking the words aloud may help you with this mourning need. Learning to say, "I have _____ cancer" to friends, family members, and even strangers when the need arises will help you come to terms with the reality of your diagnosis and prognosis.

- At times you may push away the reality of your cancer. This is normal and necessary for your survival. You will come to integrate the reality in doses as you are ready.

CARPE DIEM

Maybe you've been keeping this reality from someone in your life. Today, tell this person.

9.

UNDERSTAND THE SIX NEEDS OF MOURNING

Need #2: Embrace the pain of your losses

"In the godforsaken, obscene quicksand of life, there is a deafening alleluia rising from the souls of those who weep, and of those who weep with those who weep. If you watch, you will see the hand of God putting the stars back in their skies one by one."

— Ann Weems

- This need requires people with cancer to embrace the pain of their losses—something we naturally don't want to do. It is easier to avoid, repress, or push away the pain. It is in embracing your grief, however, that you will learn to reconcile yourself to it.

- In the early days after your diagnosis, your pain may seem ever-present. Your every thought and feeling, every moment of every day, may seem consumed by painful thoughts and feelings about your diagnosis and prognosis. During this time, you will probably need to seek refuge from your pain now and then. Go for a walk, read a book, watch TV, talk to supportive friends and family about the normal things of everyday life.

- Despite what you may have heard, acknowledging the pain is not about "feeling sorry for yourself"; it is about being honest about how cancer is impacting your life.

- While you do need to embrace the pain of your losses from cancer, you must do it in doses, over time. You simply cannot take in the enormity of loss all at once. It's healthy to seek distractions and allow yourself bits of pleasure each day.

CARPE DIEM

If you feel up to it, allow yourself a time for embracing pain today. Dedicate 15 minutes to thinking about and feeling your losses from cancer. Reach out to someone who doesn't try to take your pain away and spend some time with him.

10.

UNDERSTAND THE SIX
NEEDS OF MOURNING

Need #3: Remember your past

"In a sense, having cancer takes you by the shoulders and shakes you."
— Elizabeth Edwards

- Your life story began long before your cancer diagnosis. Yes, cancer is now part of your life story, but remembering your past makes hoping for your future possible.

- Cancer is a wake-up call. To embrace how it fits into your life and to consider what your life is all about, you must take some time to reflect on your life so far. Who are you? What made you who you are? Which experiences and relationships most shaped you? Whom do you love? Which places do you love?

- During the months following my diagnosis, I found myself drawn to places that nurtured me and made me feel safe. Interestingly, I found my home to be my "safe place." In my case, I guess Dorothy was right…there's no place like home.

- Many people with cancer naturally find themselves reminiscing and wanting to reconnect with former friends and old haunts. (That's because remembering your past is a mourning need!) When we as humans experience threats to our safety, we instinctively go backward. When you have these urges and moments of remembering, take the time to slow down and really explore them. If you want to get in touch with old friends, do. Now. Don't put it off. You may be surprised at the support they can provide you with.

CARPE DIEM
Get out some old photos today and spend at least half an hour reminiscing. Share the stories and photos with someone who didn't know you then. Better yet, share them with someone who did.

11.

UNDERSTAND THE SIX NEEDS OF MOURNING

Need #4: Incorporate cancer into your self-identity

"Not until we are lost do we begin to understand ourselves."
— Henry David Thoreau

- You have cancer. Coming to terms with the fact that you are someone who has cancer, or is a cancer survivor, is one of your needs of mourning.

- Cancer is scary and bad. While you might ultimately feel that cancer is something that has given you gifts (more on that later in this book), you probably wish that cancer wasn't the price you had to pay. In short, cancer is a part of your self-identity that you wish weren't.

- But whether you like it or not, cancer became a significant part of your life's journey. Like other life challenges, such as a history of abuse, a disability, or bad choices, cancer is one aspect of who you are. No, cancer does not define you. But it is a part of who you have become. You need to re-anchor yourself, to reconstruct your self-identity. This is arduous and painful work.

- While you must work through this difficult need yourself, I can assure you that many people with cancer ultimately learn to not only accept but embrace this new part of themselves.

CARPE DIEM

Write out a response to this prompt: I used to be _____.
Since my cancer diagnosis, I am _____. This makes me
feel _____. Keep writing as long as you want.

12.

UNDERSTAND THE SIX
NEEDS OF MOURNING

Need #5: Search for meaning

*"Because there is no glory in illness. There is no meaning to it.
There is no honor in dying of it."*

— John Green

• When we are diagnosed with a life-threatening illness, we naturally question the meaning and purpose of life and death.

• "Why" questions may surface uncontrollably and often precede "How" questions. "Why did this have to happen?" and "Why me?" come before "How will I live my remaining years as well as I can?"

• Sometimes we are taught, "Don't ask why. It doesn't do you any good." Yet it is natural to ask why and search for meaning.

• You will almost certainly question your philosophy of life and explore religious and spiritual values as you work on this need.

• Remember that having faith or spirituality does not negate your need to mourn. Even if you believe in an afterlife of some kind, your life here on Earth has still been affected by cancer. It's normal to feel dumbfounded and angry at a God whom you may feel has permitted such a thing to happen.

• Ultimately, you may decide that there is no answer to the question "Why did this happen?" Especially in this age of modern medicine, cancer does not make sense. It never will.

CARPE DIEM
Write down a list of "Why" questions that have surfaced for you since your diagnosis. Find a friend or counselor who will explore these questions with you without thinking she has to give you answers.

13.

UNDERSTAND THE SIX NEEDS OF MOURNING

Need #6: Receive ongoing support from others

"When someone has cancer, the whole family and everyone who loves them does, too."

— Terri Clark

• As mourners, we need the support of others if we are to heal.

• Don't feel ashamed by your dependence on others right now. If you are still undergoing treatment, you may need a lot of help. You may need someone to take you to and from appointments and to accompany you to treatment sessions. You may need help running errands, doing laundry, caring for children, or paying bills. Don't feel bad about this. Instead, take comfort knowing that others care.

• Unfortunately, our society places too much value on "carrying on" and "doing well." So, many people with cancer are abandoned by their friends and family soon after the diagnosis or early treatment. We hope this did not happen to you, but if it did, know that many cancer survivors share your experience.

• Other cancer survivors can be an excellent source of social, emotional, and spiritual support. They "get it." Consider joining a support group.

• Grief is experienced in "doses" over months and years, not quickly and efficiently, and you will need the continued support of your friends and family for a long time. If you are not getting this support, ask for it. Usually people are more than willing to help—they just don't have any idea what to do (and what not to do).

CARPE DIEM

Sometimes your friends want to support you but don't know *how.*
Ask! Call your closest friend right now and tell him you need his help
through the coming weeks and months.

14.

PRACTICE PATIENCE

"Why is patience so important?"
"Because it makes us pay attention."

— Paulo Coelho

- I'm sure you've realized by now that the cancer journey is often long and uncertain. And because your cancer experience becomes part of who you are, it never really, totally, ever goes away.

- In our hurry-up North American culture, patience can be especially hard to come by. We have all been conditioned to believe that if we want something, we should be able to get it instantly. But cancer diagnosis and treatment doesn't work like that. And cancer itself usually doesn't respond like that.

- And so, you must learn to be patient. Be patient with yourself. Be patient with your care team. Be patient with your friends and family. You are doing the best you can, as are they.

- Practicing patience means relinquishing control. Just as you cannot truly control your cancer, you cannot control your cancer grief. Yes, you can set your intention to embrace your grief and take steps to mourn well, and these practices will certainly serve you well on your journey, but you cannot control the particulars of what life will continue to lay before you.

CARPE DIEM
When you are feeling impatient, silently repeat this phrase: I am here.
I am now. You are here. You are now. May God bless us both.

15.

UNDERSTAND WHAT IT MEANS TO BE "TRAUMATIZED"

"Anxiety is a thin stream of fear trickling through the mind. If encouraged, it cuts a channel into which all other thoughts are drained."

— Arthur Somers Roche

- Depending on the circumstances of your diagnosis and treatment, you may have been traumatized by cancer. The word "traumatize" comes from the Greek words meaning "wound" and "pierce." You have sustained a significant psychological and perhaps physical wound, and your mind and soul have been wounded by the experience.

- In this sense, the word "trauma" also refers to the intense feelings of shock, fear, anxiety, and helplessness that are sometimes part of the experience of cancer diagnosis and treatment. Trauma is caused by events of such intensity of emotion or fear that they activate our bodies' primitive fight-or-flight responses.

- After a traumatic experience, our brains sometimes get stuck in the fight-or-flight response. We might continue to have upsetting thoughts about the surgery, the biopsy, or the doctor's appointment when we received the diagnosis. We might feel ongoing numbness, irritability, fear, and anxiety.

- A sudden, unexpected medical diagnosis can create a kind of psychic injury. So can a traumatic treatment or hospital experience. If any part of your cancer experience has felt traumatic, your cancer grief may be especially complicated.

CARPE DIEM
If you have been having frightening or intrusive thoughts about your diagnosis and treatment, share them with someone else today.

16.

NURTURE HOPE

"The joy is that we can take back our bodies, reclaim our health, and restore ourselves to balance. We can take power over how and what we eat. We can rejuvenate and recharge ourselves, bringing healing to the wounds we carry inside us, and bringing to fuller life the wonderful person that each of us has become."

— John Robbins

- Those who have gone through the dark night of a cancer diagnosis and treatment would want us to give you one simple message: You *will* endure and move through this ordeal.

- If your diagnosis is recent, you may think you cannot get through this. You can and you will. There may even come a day when the cancer is not the first thing you think of when you wake up in the morning.

- Sometimes people with cancer struggle with feeling that maybe they don't even want to survive, that they cannot go through another surgery or another round of treatment. Only you can say for sure how much is too much. But a week or a month from now, you may well find yourself feeling that life is worth living again. For now, think of how important you are to your children or grandchildren, your partner, your parents, your siblings, and your friends.

- Nurturing hope sometimes means living with trust in whatever comes.

CARPE DIEM

Create a vision board for your future. Grab a stack of old magazines and newspapers and cut out images that represent your hopes and dreams. Include a photo of yourself and your loved ones on your vision board, since remembering your past and continuing to love the important people in your life will also be part of your future. Hang this vision board where you will see it often.

17.

BE KIND TO YOUR BODY

"Take care of your body. It's the only place you have to live."
— John Rohn

- As you have probably discovered, just the diagnosis of cancer, let alone the treatment, can take a toll on your body. Do you feel tension in your body right now?

- The physical symptoms of grief and anxiety—including physical and emotional exhaustion, uncontrollable crying, trouble sleeping, heart palpitations, headaches, and more—can compound the physical effects of cancer and its treatment.

- Your stress and grief may also worsen any chronic conditions you had before your diagnosis, such as high blood pressure, eczema, asthma, or depression. Understandably, you may also be distracted by the events of the diagnosis and treatment of your cancer and forget to take needed medicines. If this happens, your physical condition may worsen dangerously.

- Nurturing your body during this time is essential. You may have to take a step back, slow down, and focus on your physical needs. You may need to take time away from work or routine demands. You must be kind to yourself by supplying your body with the good nutrition, water, rest, and exercise it needs.

CARPE DIEM
Do at least one nice thing for your body today. Consider a walk, a healthy meal, a warm cup of tea, or simply a hot bath.

18.

EXPRESS YOUR SPIRITUALITY

"Above all, cancer is a spiritual practice that teaches me about faith and resilience."

— Kris Carr

• Above all, grief is a spiritual journey of the heart and soul. Illness and loss invite you to consider why people live, why people die, and what gives life meaning and purpose. These are the most spiritual questions we have language to form.

• You can discover spiritual understanding in many ways and through many practices—prayer, worship, and meditation among them. You can nurture your spirituality in many places—nature, church, temple, mosque, monastery, retreat center, or kitchen table. No one can "give" you spirituality from the outside in. Even when you gain spiritual understanding from a specific faith tradition, the understanding is yours alone, discovered through self-examination, reflection, and spiritual transformation.

• Mourning invites you down a spiritual path at once similar to that of others yet simultaneously your own. The reality that you have picked up this book shows that you are seeking to understand and embrace your cancer grief. Sometimes this happens within a faith tradition through its scriptures, community of believers, and teachers. Other times a book is just what you need to support and gently guide you in ways that bring comfort and hope.

CARPE DIEM

If you attend a place of worship, visit it today, either for services or an informal time of prayer and solitude. If you don't have a place of worship, perhaps you have a friend who seems spiritually grounded. Ask her how she learned to nurture her spirituality. Sometimes, someone else's ideas and practices provide just what you need to stimulate your own spiritual self-care.

19.

SCHEDULE SOMETHING THAT GIVES YOU PLEASURE EACH AND EVERY DAY

"I'm dying and I'm having fun. And I'm going to keep having fun every day I have left. Because there's no other way to play."
— Randy Pausch

• When we're in the middle of cancer treatment, it can be hard to get out of bed in the morning. We're tired, we feel crappy, and we're emotionally drained.

• Part of my early experience with cancer was anhedonia, which is a clinical term that therapists sometimes use to describe the flatness of depression. *An* means "without" and *hedonia* means "pleasure."

• To counterbalance your normal and necessary physical challenges and grief, and to fight anhedonia, purposefully plan something you enjoy doing into every day.

• Reading, baking, going for a walk, having lunch with a friend, playing computer games—whatever brings you enjoyment.

• Make a "things that make me happy" tote bag. Gather up some items that are or represent activities you enjoy: a book, a movie, your favorite teabags, your knitting, a chocolate bar, crossword puzzles, your iPad, a small photo album, a list of the phone numbers of three friends who always make you feel better whenever you talk to them. Keep this tote bag handy in the coming months, whether you're at home or in the hospital or at the doctor's office for treatment.

CARPE DIEM
Put together your happy bag today. If you're not feeling up to it, ask someone to help you.

20.

LEARN TO CHECK IN WITH YOURSELF

"To array a man's will against his sickness is the supreme art of medicine."

— Henry Ward Beecher

- How are you feeling? When you have cancer, a question that used to be so simple can now seem extremely complex. So, how *are* you feeling, right this minute? Learn to quickly check in with yourself physically, emotionally, socially, cognitively, and spiritually.

- Use your mind to scan your body from head to toe. Do you hurt anywhere? Are you tense anywhere? Are you cold? Hungry? Nauseous? Stop what you are doing and take time to address your physical needs.

- How are you feeling emotionally? Identify your feelings and share them with someone.

- Take your social temperature. Do you feel like company? Is there someone you miss whom you could call or visit? Or do you need to retreat to your bedroom for some solitude?

- How are you doing cognitively? Are you thinking clearly, or are you distracted or discombobulated?

- Take a moment to take your spiritual pulse as well. If your spirit feels muted or extinguished, stop whatever you are doing and take a five-minute spirit break. (See Idea 67.)

CARPE DIEM
This very moment, check in with all five aspects of your being. Then attend to the one that needs attention the most.

21.

MAKE AN INVENTORY OF SURVIVAL STRATEGIES

"It is necessary to develop a strategy that utilizes all the physical conditions and elements that are directly at hand. The best strategy relies upon an unlimited set of responses."

— Morihei Ueshiba

• What has helped you cope with stress and loss in the past? These strategies will probably help you now, too. Use your cognitive skills to think through and strategize a plan to deal with the stress of cancer.

• Make a list of the most difficult times in your life and the ways in which you helped yourself live through them. Did you spend time with family? Turn to your faith? Help take care of someone else? How did you take care of your body? Can you make use of any of these survival techniques today?

• Knowing what calms you is also important. Getting a massage, taking a walk, going for a swim, talking to your sister on the phone, walking the dog, meditating—find what works for you.

CARPE DIEM

Make a list of what you need to get through in the next month. Ask your friends and family to help you do everything that needs doing.

22.

EAT WELL TO STAY STRONG

"I believe wholeheartedly in my diet as a means of helping my body minimize the risk of cancer recurrence. I now look at everything I eat in a very mindful way, asking myself, 'How does this food nourish me? How does it promote my recovery?' By asking myself these questions, I am acknowledging that food nourishes both the body and the soul."

— Diane Dyers, M.S, R.D.

- Because cancer treatments affect healthy cells as well as cancer cells, it is important to give your body the tools it needs to rebuild and stay strong. In the past, doctors often told cancer patients to eat anything that sounded good, just to keep their weight on, but it really does matter which foods you eat.

- Try nausea busters. The Chinese have used ginger as a nausea remedy for 2,000 years. Use fresh ginger in stir-fries, soups, and tea, or sprinkle powdered ginger over melon or rice. Whole-wheat toast helps settle nausea and keeps your digestive tract healthy, too.

- Increase protein. Making sure you get the right kind of protein is essential in keeping your strength up. Almond butter is a delicious source of protein (five grams in one serving) and contains benzaldehyde, which research shows to be toxic to cancer cells. Lentils, a pint-sized powerhouse, pack nine grams of protein and almost eight grams of fiber in each serving.

- Include strength builders. Garlic is loaded with allicin, which has been shown to destroy cancer cells, reduce the rate of cell division, and support the immune system. Spinach is rich in folates, which helps your body build healthy cells. It is also a great source of lutein, an antioxidant that may significantly reduce the incidence of cancer.

CARPE DIEM
Look for recipes that include some of these superfoods. Include them in your diet daily.

23.

YIELD TO SILENCE AND SOLITUDE...

*"Inside myself is a place where I live all alone, and that's where
I renew my springs that never dry up."*
— Pearl Buck

- The mysteries of cancer, life, and death invite you to experience periods of silence and solitude. Have you noticed yourself craving alone time more often lately?

- Many of the normal symptoms of grief are invitations to withdraw. Numbness, confusion, and the lethargy of grief try to slow you down so you can be alone with your thoughts and feelings.

- It's painful, this lonely struggle. But it's also necessary. This is your life and yours alone. Yes, you are connected to others, but it is you who has cancer. You must decide for yourself what this means to you and how you will proceed.

- You may not have access to a cloistered monastery, a walk in the woods, or a stroll on the beach, but you do have the capacity to quiet yourself. Consciously hush yourself and place trust in the peace you help initiate. As you sit with silence, you acknowledge that you value the need to suspend, slow down, and turn inward as part of the grief journey. Giving attention to the instinct to mourn from the inside out requires that you befriend silence and respect how vital it is to your healing journey.

CARPE DIEM

Today, be silent for a while—silent with yourself and with God. For many people, this is a difficult spiritual practice, but it is also one that is well worth the effort.

24.

...BUT DO NOT WITHDRAW ALTOGETHER

"Often we can help each other most by leaving each other alone; at other times we need the hand-grasp and the word of cheer."
— Elbert Hubbard

• While silence and solitude are essential ingredients to healing your cancer grief, so is social connection. We've said that receiving and accepting support from others is one of the six needs of mourning. That's because life is really all about love.

• When we're hurt, we naturally withdraw. Like injured animals, we retreat to our caves and lick our wounds. But if we withdraw too often or for too long, we sever the ties that make life worth living. We pretend that we don't need anyone else, and, maybe worse, that they don't need us.

• If you're an introvert or someone who's prone to self-isolate anyway, you may have to force yourself to continue to nurture relationships with friends and family members in the coming weeks and months. Ask your best friend to take on the challenge of rousting you from your hiding spot at least a few times a week. Connect with people online and via e-mail.

• Look into cancer support groups, too. Even if you're not much of a talker in these types of situations, you will still benefit from the shared stories, the accepted tears, and the tangible camaraderie.

CARPE DIEM
Reach out to at least one other person today, preferably face-to-face.

25.

BE ON YOUR OWN TEAM

"As a cancer doctor, I'm looking forward to being out of a job."
— Daniel Kraft

- Cancer is a complex disease. That's why there are so many healthcare providers who are part of your care team!
- In addition to a general physician and a medical oncologist, you may have a surgeon, a radiation oncologist, oncology nurses, oncology technicians, a social worker, a psychologist, a pathologist, a rehab specialist, a dietitian, and a navigator.
- That's a lot of expertise in your corner! But never forget that *you* are also an integral part of this team.
- Learning about your cancer and piping up when you have a question or concern will make you a participant in your care instead of a mere recipient. Participating will make you feel a little more in control of a hard-to-control disease. It will also likely make your care more consistent and comprehensive.

CARPE DIEM
Ask "why?" at your next appointment. "Why am I receiving this particular chemotherapy?" or "Why am I not having radiation?" Your questions will spur your care team to ensure that they're doing their very best.

26.

BE HONEST WITH THE CHILDREN

"Sometimes you need to talk to a two-year-old just so you can understand life again."

— Author Unknown

• If you have children or grandchildren in your life, what they need and deserve most of all is your honesty. I often say that children can cope with what they know. What they cannot cope with is what they *don't* know or have never been told. Secrecy and taboos are bad for children. Open, honest, loving communication is good for children.

• Of course, what any given child can understand about cancer and stages and treatment depends on her age and developmental maturity. The important thing is to follow her lead.

• Use the word "cancer." If he asks, be honest about your prognosis— in words that he can understand. Don't scare him unnecessarily, but don't sugarcoat, either. Let his questions guide you. Say a few words, then stop and listen. Cry if you feel like crying. Hold him if you can.

• Remember that cancer is a journey, and that lots of small conversations along the way are better than one big "tell-all." Kids are often satisfied with just a little bit of information at a time. Then they need to go off and play, because play is how they process the world around them. After they've played for a while, they'll often come back with another question or thought.

• When someone they love is sick or in danger, children naturally grieve. And grieving children need the love and support of caring adults to mourn their grief. Be sure to let the other adults in your children's lives know what is happening so they can proactively support the children in the coming weeks and months.

CARPE DIEM
Ask a child in your life today if she has any questions about your illness. Answer her questions briefly, then pause to see how she reacts. Tell her you love her.

27.

LEARN TO MEDITATE

"Cancer taught me to live only in the day I'm in. In the moment I'm in. Some moments, I simply ground myself by touching the desk, the table, the wall wherever I am and say, 'You're right here. Stay put in this moment.'"

— Regina Brett

- Meditation is simply quiet, relaxed contemplation. It's a great way to ease tension and anxiety. It's also a way to get in touch with your truest thoughts and feelings.

- You needn't follow any particular rules or techniques in order to meditate. Simply find a quiet place where you can focus without distraction and rid your mind of superficial thoughts and concerns.

- Relax your muscles and close your eyes if you'd like.

- Focus on your breath. When your mind starts thinking its monkey thoughts (which it will!), return your focus to breathing in and out.

- Try meditating for 10 to 15 minutes each day. It may help center you and provide a time of respite from your cancer grief thoughts and feelings.

- If you've tried meditating in the past and have discovered that it's not a good fit for you, that's OK. Meditation isn't for everyone. Try other techniques instead.

CARPE DIEM
If you're unsure how to get started on meditating, try listening to guided audio meditations. You can find a number of free ones online, including these on the UCLA Mindful Awareness Research Center website: www.marc.ucla.edu/body.cfm?id=22.

28.

SLEEP WELL

"The nicest thing for me is sleep; then at least I can dream."
— Marilyn Monroe

• How is your sleep? Nothing is more essential to your health than restful and sufficient sleep. Yet as you battle cancer, you may not be sleeping well. In fact, one in three people has trouble falling or staying asleep even without the added stress of cancer.

• Most people average about seven-and-a-half hours of sleep a night, but with the increased fatigue and feelings of exhaustion that are common with cancer treatment, you may need more. Actually, cancer or no cancer, most of us get less sleep than we need, and studies show that most of us would sleep an hour longer if we could.

• A normal night's sleep consists of several distinct stages and types of sleep. Stage 1 is the twilight zone between being awake and asleep. Stage 2 sleep brings larger brain waves, and we are no longer conscious of our surroundings. In Stages 3 and 4, our brains produce slower and even larger waves, referred to as delta or slow-wave sleep.

• After about 90 minutes in the four stages of quiet sleep, the brain shifts into the more active stage characterized by rapid eye movement (REM). Brain waves during REM resemble those of wakefulness, but the large muscles of the body cannot move. This is the time of vivid dreaming. During a typical night we spend about 25 percent of the time in REM sleep and may have four or five cycles of REM sleep.

• In today's busy world, we often do not leave enough time in our lives for adequate sleep, and many people start the day off tired and run down. Especially as you battle cancer, it is essential to get the sleep you need.

CARPE DIEM

If you are not sleeping well, talk to your physician about your sleep troubles. She may have excellent sleep suggestions for people with cancer. She may also prescribe a sleep aid.

29.

ENJOY GREEN TEA

"Tea began as a medicine and grew into a beverage."
— Kakuzo Okakura

- The Chinese have known about the medicinal effects of green tea since ancient times. It has been used to treat many physical ailments for more than 4,000 years. Ever since its discovery, its cultivation and consumption have been encouraged because of its apparent ability to ward off disease, strengthen powers of concentration, cleanse the body, and aid digestion. Centuries later, modern research has begun to confirm many of those early beliefs.

- Studies have proven that green tea has positive effects on the immune system and reduces infection rates. It has also been shown to help prevent heart disease by lowering bad cholesterol (LDL), raising good cholesterol (HDL), and inhibiting the formation of clots that cause strokes and heart attacks. It even slows cancer cell growth.

- The secret of green tea is in the powerful antioxidants it contains. Other types of tea lack these beneficial chemicals.

- Green tea can provide you with a basic health boost during your treatment. The simple act of drinking tea daily can also be a mind-clearing ritual. Green tea has long been used in tea ceremonies throughout Asia for its calming effects.

- Try adding green tea, hot or cold, to your life. This simple act will help care for your mind and body and add a reassuring ritual to your life.

CARPE DIEM

Start a daily regimen of taking time to relax, clear your mind, and enjoy a cup of warm, soothing green tea. Let it rejuvenate you.

30.

MOURN HAIR LOSS, TOO

"When I look in the mirror bald, I can be overwhelmed by my strength or disarmed by my vulnerability. There are moments when I see a warrior, a fighter, a bad-ass. Then there are moments when I see a cancer patient, a victim, or a shadow of my former self. I am learning to accept, embrace, and love my many selves."

— Jenna Benn

- Hair loss can be a traumatic part of cancer loss because it affects your self-image. Your cancer treatments may cause some or all of your hair to fall out. It may come out in clumps in the shower or as you brush, or you may find it in bunches on the pillow in the morning.

- Almost everyone is distressed about this change in body image. After all—it's bad enough that you have a life-threatening disease and you may feel awful from the treatments. Losing your hair only adds insult to injury. What's more, it announces to the world: I have cancer!— something you may not want to share with strangers.

- If you think you may want a wig, consider buying it before treatment begins. Get a prescription for the wig since it may be covered by insurance. Go shopping for turbans, hats, or scarves with a friend.

- If you're sad or angry about your hair loss, talk to someone about it. Sharing your thoughts and feelings with other cancer patients who've experienced hair loss may give you a new perspective.

CARPE DIEM

Consider cutting your hair short before it starts falling out. Also, the American Cancer Society provides free wigs to cancer patients. Call your local office to learn more.

31.

VISUALIZE

"As you think, so shall you become."
— Bruce Lee

- Indulge us as we start this Idea with a silly reference. In the very funny book and movie *The Princess Bride*, the hero, Westley, is captured and tortured by the evil Count Rugen. (It's funny, we promise!) Strapped to the torture Machine, Westley is able to endure the pain because he "takes his mind away." That is, he has trained himself to think of his beloved Princess Buttercup whenever his reality is unpleasant.

- The power of visualization can in fact do incredible things. In one study, the muscles of people who lifted weights were compared to the muscles of people who simply visualized lifting weights. The muscle mass of the actual weight lifters increased 30 percent, but the muscle mass of the visualizers also increased—by 13.5 percent.

- How can you use this to your advantage during your cancer treatment and beyond? Visualize your desired outcome. Picture yourself healthy and healed. Flesh out this image with as many details as possible. Where are you? What are you wearing? What does it feel like? Smell like? Taste like? Who else is there?

- During unpleasant experiences, such as surgical recovery or chemo, try visualizing your happy place. If you could, where would you go to relax and be joyful? Go there in your imagination by "taking your mind away."

- As with any skill, visualizing improves with practice. And you can practice visualization anytime, anywhere, on your cancer journey.

CARPE DIEM
Today, visualize the cancer outcome you desire. Set an alarm and practice for five minutes. Do this every day, and see if you can work yourself up to 10 or 15 minutes at a time.

32.

BREAK THE SILENCE

"My silences had not protected me. Your silence will not protect you. But for every real word spoken, for every attempt I had ever made to speak those truths for which I am still seeking, I had made contact with other women while we examined the words to fit a world in which we all believed, bridging our differences."

— Audre Lorde

- Grief is silent. It's your inner thoughts and feelings about your cancer. And while those thoughts and feelings can be very loud and demanding inside you, they are soundless outside you.

- The silence of grief belies its violence. It doesn't feel very meek and calm and quiet inside you, does it?

- To heal your grief, you must give it voice. You must find ways to break the silence.

- Here's another way to think of it: Your grief is a significant part of your inner truth right now. For you to live congruently, it must also be part of your outer truth. Living congruently means that your words, actions, and deeds match up with your thoughts, beliefs, and passions. You do what you believe. You act as you think. You say what's on your mind.

CARPE DIEM

Today, share a powerful aspect of your cancer grief that you so far have not shared. What worry or anxiety has been silently consuming you? Tell it to someone else.

33.

MOVE

"It's helpful to realize that this very body that we have, that's sitting right here right now…with its aches and its pleasures…is exactly what we need to be fully human, fully awake, fully alive."

— Pema Chodron

- We all know how important physical activity is to our physical health, but did you know that it also has a significant effect on your mood? Research shows that exercise helps lift anxiety and ease depression.

- During your treatment period, you will almost certainly feel tired. No wonder! Your body is under assault from the inside as well as the outside. And feelings of grief and loss compound fatigue. Lay your body down three times a day for at least 20 minutes.

- But when you're able, forcing yourself to get moving every day will help you feel better.

- I often tell mourners that they need to put their grief into motion by expressing it. This movement of thoughts and feelings is what creates opportunity for positive change. Similarly, moving your body creates physical and biochemical change that supports physical as well as emotional/spiritual healing.

CARPE DIEM
Get at least half an hour of physical activity today if you're up to it—more if your fitness level is high. You don't need to go to a gym! Gardening, housework, and all kinds of everyday activities count.

34.

KEEP DOWN EXCESS WEIGHT

"More die in the United States of too much food than of too little."
— John Kenneth Galbraith

- Cancer is a multistep process. It starts with a mutation of genetic material, then its growth is promoted by other factors. Excess abdominal fat may act like a cancer promoter.

- Fat cells act like endocrine cells, constantly producing a variety of hormones and other growth factors, called *cytokines*, into the blood stream. As a result, an overweight person's cells are urged to grow and divide at an accelerated rate. This can promote the accelerated growth of cancer cells if they are present.

- According to an American Cancer Society study, there is a direct relationship between the amount of excess weight and the risk of death from most cancers. You may carry risk factors for cancer that you can't do anything about, such as age, gender, or family history, but weight is a risk factor that you can do something about.

- Reducing excess weight doesn't just reduce your risk of future cancers; it can also increase your chances of survival by reducing the promotion of cancer cell growth.

CARPE DIEM
Talk to your doctor about your body mass index (BMI) and ask if your current weight is appropriate.

35.

TAKE A DEEP BREATH

"All the principles of heaven and earth are living inside you. Life itself is truth, and this will never change. Everything in heaven and earth breathes. Breath is the thread that ties creation together."

— Moriehei Ueshiba

- A very basic need of survival is the air we breathe. With the stress of your cancer losses, even breathing may seem difficult. If you are anxious, you may be taking rapid, short, shallow breaths, which may cause you to feel lightheaded or dizzy.

- Simply taking a deep breath can trigger a natural relaxation response within your body. Breathing slowly and deeply is one way to "turn off " your stress reaction and "turn on" relaxation.

- By inhaling deeply and allowing your lungs to take in as much oxygen as possible, you can begin to relieve your tension. Best of all, deep breathing can be done anywhere and anytime.

- First, sit or stand and place your hands on your stomach. Inhale slowly and deeply through your nose, letting your stomach expand as much as possible. Many people are "backward breathers" and tighten their stomachs when breathing in. But by placing your hands on your stomach, you can actually feel when you are breathing properly, which will help trigger relaxation. When you have breathed in as much as possible, hold your breath for a few seconds before exhaling.

- With your hands still on your stomach, exhale slowly through your mouth, pursing your lips like you are going to whistle. By pursing your lips, you can control how fast you exhale and keep your airways open as long as possible. When your lungs feel empty, start the cycle again by inhaling and exhaling. Repeat this at least three or four times per session. See how much calmer you feel already.

CARPE DIEM
Practice deep breathing for a few minutes three or four times daily, or whenever you begin to feel tense.

36.

KNOW THAT YOU ARE LOVED

"Friendship is unnecessary, like philosophy, like art... It has no survival value; rather it is one of those things which give value to survival."
— C.S. Lewis

• As Jane Howard wisely observed, "Call it a clan, call it a network, call it a tribe, call it a family. Whatever you call it, whoever you are, you need one." Yes, love from family, friends, and community gives life meaning and purpose. Look around for expressions of care and concern. These are people who love you and want to support you.

• Some of those who love you may not know how to reach out to you, but they still love you. Reflect on the people who care about you and the ways in which your life matters. Open your heart and have gratitude for those who love you.

• In contrast, if you lose this connection, you suffer alone and in isolation. You feel disconnected from the world around you. Feeling pessimistic, you may retreat even more. You begin to sever your relationships and make your world smaller. You may even convince yourself you are a victim and continue to separate yourself from the need for community.

• It is vital to create a sense of community that is spiritually nurturing and responsive to your needs during your cancer journey. Your relationships with family, friends, and community are connected like a circle, with no end and no beginning. When you allow yourself to be a part of that circle, you find your place. You realize you belong and are a vital part of a bigger whole.

CARPE DIEM
Get out some notes, cards, or e-mails you have received from people who care about you. Re-read them and remind yourself that you are loved. Then, call someone you love and express gratitude that she or he is in your life.

37.

SET YOUR INTENTION ON OPTIMISM

"Choose to be optimistic. It feels better."
— Dalai Lama XIV

• You aren't in total control of your life. Cancer has taught you that.

• But you can control the attitude with which you live your life. You choose whether you intend to experience spiritual pessimism or spiritual optimism. For example, if you choose to believe that God is vengeful and punishes us for our sins by causing illness and death, it will be next to impossible for you to make it through difficult times. Not only will you carry the pain of your losses from cancer, but you will also carry the guilt and blame of being so sinful that you deserved cancer in your life.

• By contrast, if you set your intention to be what I would call "spiritually optimistic" and believe that looking for the love and the good and the beauty of each day is a wonderful way to live, then you will experience much more joy and happiness.

• Same circumstances, different experience.

• You might tell yourself, "I can and will reach out for support during my cancer journey. I will become filled with hope that I can experience joy each and every day." Together with these words, you might form mental pictures of yourself hugging and talking to your friends and enjoying the little things. Setting your intention on optimism is not only a way of getting through each day (although it is indeed that!), it is a way of guiding your grief to the best possible outcome.

CARPE DIEM

Talk to someone who knows you well (preferably an optimist!) about whether you are, generally speaking, an optimist or a pessimist. How can you move the needle toward optimism today?

38.

HONOR THE BEFORE AND THE AFTER

"All changes, even the most longed for, have their melancholy; for what we leave behind us is a part of ourselves; we must die to one life before we can enter another."

— Anatole France

- Some things that happen in life are so intensely special or traumatic that it seems like they're burned into our memories.

- You probably remember well exceptional moments such as your first kiss, your wedding day, and the birth of your babies. But you also probably can recall in vivid detail some of your most difficult experiences.

- Being diagnosed with cancer is one of those traumatic, difficult experiences that you will never forget. And thereafter, it becomes like a bookmark that divides the story of your life into Before Cancer and After Cancer.

- You know what they say—stuff happens. What happened to you is cancer. You don't have to like it. But if you acknowledge it as the significant experience it is, you will be living your truth. If you honor the impact it has on you physically, emotionally, socially, cognitively, and spiritually, if you learn to embrace the fact that the you Before Cancer is different than the you After Cancer, you will be living your truth.

CARPE DIEM
Talk to someone or journal today about how the you After Cancer is different than the you Before Cancer.

39.

DON'T BE ALARMED BY MOOD SWINGS

"Cancer is not a straight line. It's up and down."
— Elizabeth Edwards

- The cancer journey often has a lot of ups and downs. Your diagnosis and prognosis may change over time. Your treatment may leave you feeling fine one day and terrible the next. Your emotional reserves may go from depleted to replenished then back to depleted again.

- In ever-changing circumstances like these, mood swings are normal and understandable. They do not mean you're crazy.

- Still, no matter how normal mood swings might be for people with cancer, they don't feel good. It's stressful to feel yanked around by your emotions like that.

- If you're suffering from mood swings, talk to a friend about them. Find other ways to cope, too, such as meditation and physical activity. Planning how you will respond to your next mood shift will help you feel a little more prepared, a little more in control of your out-of-control life.

CARPE DIEM
Make a list of 10 things you could try the next time you're feeling yanked around by cancer.

40.

BEFRIEND YOUR FEAR

"Cancer is messy and scary. You throw everything at it, but don't forget to throw love at it. It turns out that might be the best weapon of all."
— Regina Brett

- Facing the prospect of death, especially a premature death, is understandably very scary. It's scary for you as an individual, and it's scary for you on behalf of those who depend on you. That is why fear is often a natural and necessary part of cancer grief.

- Some say that fear is a vestige of our evolutionary drive to survive. For humans, it wasn't that long ago that our ancestors had to battle daily for safety, shelter, and food. Our innate fight-or-flight response kept us alive. We modern humans still possess this "lizard-brain" fear response, even though we no longer live in a world in which we are in imminent danger each day.

- You can choose to befriend your fear by exploring it instead of suppressing it. What are you afraid of? Talk about your fears with someone else. Write about them in your journal. Share them in the safety of a cancer support group.

- Try to not be afraid of your fear. It is your friend because it is giving you valuable information: what you are most afraid of tells you what is most important to you. And identifying what is most important to you can help you live each and every precious day you have left on this Earth—whether that is weeks or decades—to the fullest.

CARPE DIEM
Answer this question: What am I most afraid of right now and why?
Try to be specific. Talk to someone about this fear today.

41.

IF YOU FEEL HELPLESS, TALK ABOUT IT

"Grief is a most peculiar thing; we're so helpless in the face of it. It's like a window that will simply open of its own accord. The room grows cold, and we can do nothing but shiver."

— Arthur Golden

- People with cancer often feel helpless. After all, defective cells took hold in your body and started colonizing. This is or was literally happening inside you, without your permission. If you feel helpless, it's no wonder!

- With cancer, the process of diagnosis and treatment can be extremely involved and time-consuming. How many doctors' appointments and procedures have you been through so far? The medical (and financial) rigmarole can make you feel helpless too. It may seem like you're pinballing from one office or piece of paperwork to the next.

- Of course, the ultimate helplessness in cancer stems from the hard-to-swallow fact that we are not in complete control of our own lives and our own destinies.

- If you feel helpless since your diagnosis, talk to someone about your thoughts and feelings. Sharing your most powerful, prominent inside feelings outside of yourself takes away some of their power. Mourning eases what's inside you.

CARPE DIEM

Today, talk to someone about your feelings of helplessness. After this conversation, notice if your sense of powerlessness has softened, if only a tiny little bit.

42.

IF YOU FEEL ANGRY, TALK ABOUT IT

"Anger is a symptom, a way of cloaking and expressing feelings too awful to experience directly—hurt, bitterness, grief, and, most of all, fear."

— Joan Rivers

- Anger is a common and understandable response after a cancer diagnosis.
- *It's not fair!* we think. *I'm too young!* or *I've taken good care of myself!* or *I have too many people counting on me!*
- After a cancer diagnosis and throughout the course of treatment, sometimes our anger gets directed at a certain person, such as a doctor, or at an entity, such as an insurance company. We can also feel angry with others for what we perceive someone did or did not do that may have contributed to our illness.
- Sometimes those of us with cancer feel angry with ourselves. If we put off diagnostic testing, for example, or ignored early symptoms, we might feel like the only one to blame is ourselves.
- Anger, rage, and blame are, at bottom, protest emotions. They are how we protest a reality that we wish were not true. As with all feelings in grief, anger is neither good nor bad, right nor wrong. It simply is. And it needs to be expressed in order to be worked through.
- With anger, it's important that its expression does not physically or emotionally hurt someone else (or even ourselves). Find more neutral ways to express anger, such as intense physical activity or talking with a friend or counselor.

CARPE DIEM

Are you angry about your cancer? If you are, share your angry thoughts and feelings with a neutral but compassionate friend today.

43.

IF YOU FEEL GUILTY, TALK ABOUT IT

"Maybe there's more we all could have done, but we just have to let the guilt remind us to do better next time."

— Veronica Roth

- Sometimes people with cancer feel guilty about their own disease or circumstances.

- You might blame yourself for skipping screening tests or putting off doctors' visits. You might feel ashamed that something you did or did not do contributed to your illness, which is now also having an effect on those who love and depend on you.

- Guilt and feelings of regret might also arise if you are not feeling well enough to work right now or take care of other responsibilities.

- As with all other feelings in grief, guilt, regret, and shame are not right or wrong—they simply are. And whenever you have a feeling inside, you simply need to express it on the outside.

- Expressing your difficult thoughts and feelings is rather magical. It doesn't make them instantly disappear, but it does help soften them. And sharing them with empathetic listeners elicits understanding and often reveals new insights and, sometimes, self-forgiveness.

CARPE DIEM

Silently, to yourself, name one thing that you feel a twinge of guilt or regret about, whether it has to do with your cancer or not. Now go and share that thought with someone who cares about you.

44.

IF YOU FEEL STUCK, TALK ABOUT IT

*"The goal is to live a full, productive life even with all that ambiguity.
No matter what happens, whether the cancer never flares up again or
whether you die, the important thing is that the days that you have had
you will have lived."*

— Gilda Radner

- Cancer has a way of putting life on hold. While the Earth keeps spinning and the lives of those around you go on as usual, your reality may have you feeling trapped in the quicksand of your illness.

- The reality is that treatment may consume your life for a while. While those of us with cancer never want to "become" our cancer, we can't help but be taken over by the many appointments and tests and therapies, at least for a time.

- None of us likes the feeling of being stuck. But the truth is, your heart and soul know that you need to be stuck. You need to press the pause button and spend time embracing what is happening to you. I call it "sitting in your wound." When you sit in the wound of your grief, you surrender to it. You acquiesce to the instinct to slow down and turn inward. You allow yourself to appropriately wallow in the pain. You shut the world out for a time so that, eventually, you have created space to let the world back in.

- Sometimes feelings of aimlessness or ineffectiveness also arise. Even after your initial treatment course, you may find yourself unable to focus, to concentrate, to get anything done. Your brain is still trying to understand and process what happened. It's a form of post-traumatic stress, really. If this is happening to you, know that it's normal and that your cognitive challenges are simply a symptom telling you that you need to be patient with yourself and allow yourself to mourn.

CARPE DIEM
If you feel stuck or aimless right now, tell a friend
about your experience.

45.

EAT DESSERT FIRST...AND LAST

"Seize the moment. Remember all those women on the Titanic who waved off the dessert cart."
— Erma Bombeck

- You've probably heard this saying before. "Eat dessert first" means you shouldn't put off what you enjoy most. Instead, you should seize the moment and do what brings you joy as often as you can.

- People living with cancer often get good at eating dessert first. They quickly learn to embrace what matters to them and ignore the rest.

- On a day-to-day basis, what is your "dessert"? What gives you joy? Conversely, what things do you have to do even though you really don't like to do them? For every "have to," try doing one "love to" before and one "love to" after. Make a joy sandwich!

- For example, maybe you love pedicures and fresh flowers but you don't enjoy cleaning the kitchen. Go get a pedicure then give the kitchen a quick once-over in your lovely bare feet. Then pick or buy some fresh flowers and place them in a vase on your kitchen table.

CARPE DIEM
Plan to make at least one joy sandwich each day for the next week.

46.

MAKE LOVE A HABIT

"We are what we repeatedly do. Excellence, then, is not an act, but a habit."

— Aristotle

- Have you heard that it takes 21 days to make a new behavior a habit? The science behind the 21-day marker is rather iffy, but researchers do agree that if you continue to do something every day, eventually it becomes automatic and you no longer have to consciously *try* to do it. Instead, the activity becomes an easy, simple, mindless act. In other words, a habit.

- We believe that love is why we're here. Giving and receiving love is what makes life worth living. But how much of our daily lives do we devote to acts of love and kindness?

- Make love a habit by adding new kindness rituals to your daily routine. Kiss your spouse or partner every morning. Hug your children or friends. Write a note or email of gratitude every night before you go to sleep.

CARPE DIEM

Add one "love habit" to your daily schedule. Set a reminder in your phone or make a note to yourself on paper so you won't forget.

47.

HOLD THAT HUG FOR 20 SECONDS

"Hugs are the universal medicine."
— Author Unknown

- Human touch is powerful. Physically connecting with another human being makes us feel connected emotionally, socially, and spiritually as well.

- Recently researchers learned that longer hugs cause measurable biochemical responses. When you hug someone else for at least 20 seconds, your brain releases a hormone called *oxytocin*. Oxytocin, also called the "bonding hormone or the "love hormone," makes you feel happy and helps bond you to the person you've hugged.

- Holding hands for at least 20 seconds generates the same biochemical response.

- You'll probably want to save these long embraces for the people you're closest to. But when you do hug them or hold their hands, slowly and silently count to 20 or more and see if you notice the flush of feelings of love.

CARPE DIEM
Give someone you love a 20-second (or longer) hug today. Notice how you feel afterward.

48.

GET FAMILIAR WITH ONLINE RESOURCES

"Knowledge is power, community is strength, and positive attitude is everything."
— Lance Armstrong

- There's a lot of cancer information on the web—so much, in fact, that it's easy to get overwhelmed. But if you're trying to learn more about your cancer and treatment, it's all there, at your fingertips, free of charge, 24/7.

- The American Cancer Society's website, www.cancer.org, offers extensive, trustworthy cancer information to both those with cancer and those who care about them.

- The Association of Cancer Online Resources, or www.acor.org, is a clearinghouse for different cancer communities. If you join their multiple myeloma group, for example, you'll be welcomed into a group of nearly 2,000 people affected by that type of cancer—all of whom share ideas, answer one another's questions, and generally support one another. Similar sites include www.cancercompass.com, www.cancerforums.net, and the discussion boards that are part of www.cancer.org.

- Information sharing sites such as www.caringbridge.org can be a great way to keep a large or far-flung group of family and friends up-to-date on your treatment and health. You can start a Caring Bridge page for yourself, or someone else can do it for you. Never underestimate the power of the Internet in keeping you connected with all the people who care about you!

CARPE DIEM
Today, check out at least one of the online cancer communities mentioned in the third bullet, above. See if you might benefit from some online support and supporting.

49.
FIND NEW WAYS TO BE INTIMATE

*"There's nothing more intimate in life than simply being understood.
And understanding someone else."*
— Brad Meltzer

- Cancer often throws a monkey wrench into intimacy. Your treatment may include therapies that make you feel sick and surgeries that leave you with pain or make you feel sexually undesirable. Your partner may also be struggling with sexual thoughts and feelings right now.

- If your sexual abilities or desires have diminished, allow yourself and your partner to mourn this loss. The sexual repercussions of cancer can dramatically impact your sense of identity, both individually and as a couple. If you don't openly acknowledge this loss, you may both experience the frustration and create more distance than if you talk freely about it.

- Open communication is essential. You and your partner may be assuming that you know how one another feels—but the truth is that your assumptions may be mildly—or wildly—off base. So find quiet, safe moments, regularly, to share your sexual thoughts and feelings.

- Both of you need and deserve patience and loving understanding right now. It will take time and mutual supportiveness to get through the early challenges of cancer as a couple.

- Exploring new ways to be intimate can be freeing and healing for both of you. Work as a team on this issue. Take it slow. Go on dates—times that aren't about cancer and caregiving. Nurture romance instead of sex for a while. Touch, hold hands, and stroke one another's arms or backs. Dim the lights. Focus on the sensual instead of the sexual. And don't forget to tell each other "I love you."

CARPE DIEM
Today, make it a point to be intimate with your partner throughout the day. Hug, touch, hold hands. If you're not up for sex, say so, but don't forsake closeness.

50.

KNOW THE SIGNS OF CLINICAL DEPRESSION

"We must embrace pain and burn it as fuel for our journey."
— Kenji Miyazawa

• According to the National Institute of Mental Health, symptoms of clinical depression include:
  - Difficulty concentrating, remembering details, and making decisions.
  - Fatigue and decreased energy.
  - Feelings of guilt, worthlessness, and/or helplessness.
  - Feelings of hopelessness and/or pessimism.
  - Insomnia, early-morning wakefulness, or excessive sleeping.
  - Irritability, restlessness.
  - Loss of interest in activities or hobbies you used to enjoy.
  - Overeating or appetite loss.
  - Persistent aches or pains, headaches, cramps, or digestive problems that do not ease, even with treatment.
  - Persistent sad, anxious, or "empty" feelings.
  - Thoughts of suicide or suicide attempts.

• If your feelings of self-worth are low, if you are having trouble functioning on a day-to-day basis, and certainly if you are considering suicide, please seek help right away. Anti-depressant medication or other forms of treatment may be necessary and extremely effective for you right now.

CARPE DIEM

If you think you may be suffering from clinical depression, make an appointment to talk to your primary care physician about this specifically. As you probably know all too well, cancer patients get caught up in an overwhelming whirl of medical appointments, but your depression merits its own appointment and discussion.

51.

FIND ENCOURAGING PEOPLE

"Who helps me in a hardship truly is my friend."
— Swahili proverb

- Living with cancer can be discouraging. It is not pleasant to go through the stress of a cancer diagnosis and the physical side effects of treatment. Spending time with people who support and encourage you can make all the difference in keeping your spirits up.

- With cancer, as with support for other problems, people tend to fall into the "rule of thirds." About a third of people you know will be supportive and encouraging, about a third will be neutral (not much help but at least not negative), and a third will be openly discouraging and sometimes toxic.

- With the discouragement you may have felt in dealing with your cancer, it is important for you to seek out people who will offer you encouragement and support and who will not shame, belittle, or discourage you.

- If you don't have a good support network, call your local cancer association office and learn more about resources in your community.

CARPE DIEM

In biblical times, Barnabas, whose name means "son of encouragement," earned his nickname by encouraging his friends, even when others gave up on them. Make a list of the Barnabases in your life. Reach out and spend time with them. Allow their gift of encouragement to support you in your journey through the losses of cancer.

52.

CONNECT WITH ANIMALS

"Until one has loved an animal, a part of one's soul remains unawakened."

— Anatole France

• Animals are our natural companions. In times of crisis they can steady us and bathe us in unconditional love. Animals can open our souls to the beauty of our lives. Studies show that people live longer and have more fulfilled lives when they share their lives with an animal companion.

• Pets invite you to focus on their needs and not be so overwhelmed by your own. Taking care of an animal allows you to feel needed and loved by your pet.

• There is a special feeling of being here and now when you are with your pet. They have souls, too, and most pet owners feel this soulful connection with their four-legged friends. The unconditional love a pet shows may be just what you need during this difficult time.

• My dogs were my constant companions following my prostate surgery. Sometimes even now they ride with me to my regular follow-up appointments. I'm always somewhat anxious to learn my latest test results, and my pups help calm my spirit.

CARPE DIEM
Spend time with your pet today. If you don't have one, consider visiting an animal shelter to rescue one. If the care is too much for you, spend time with a friend's pet. Feel the soulful touch of connection with a pet.

53.

TELL THE STORY, OVER AND OVER AGAIN IF YOU FEEL THE NEED

"I know now that we never get over great losses; we absorb them, and they carve us into different, often kinder, creatures. We tell the story to get them back, to capture the traces of footfalls through the snow."

— Gail Caldwell

- Acknowledging the reality of cancer is a painful, ongoing task that we accomplish in doses, over time. A vital part of healing in grief is often "telling the story" over and over again. It's as if each time you tell the story, it becomes a little more comprehensible and bearable.

- Your cancer story may begin on the day you found a lump or the moment your doctor told you the biopsy results. It might begin earlier—maybe when you first grew concerned that you carried a genetic predisposition to cancer or when a friend or family member was diagnosed.

- Find people who are willing to listen to you tell your story, over and over again if necessary, without judgment.

CARPE DIEM

Tell the story of your diagnosis and treatment to someone today in the form of a letter or e-mail. Perhaps you can write and send this letter to a friend who lives far away.

54.

IF YOU HAVE QUESTIONS, ASK THEM

"As we must account for every idle word, so must we account for every idle silence."

— Benjamin Franklin

- After a cancer diagnosis comes a tsunami of medical lingo, treatment information, and complex choices. What's more, you're often dealing with multiple doctors and care providers. It can get extremely confusing.

- You'll probably have questions, and if you do, you should be assertive enough to ask them. If you and your family don't take charge of your course of care, no one will. But how will you remember your questions and keep all the information straight?

- Making a cancer notebook is one good technique. Write your questions down. Take it with you to every appointment. Also jot down physician names and phone numbers, appointment dates and times, and maybe daily notes on any side effects you might be experiencing.

- Some health systems offer the free services of a "cancer navigator"— usually a nurse whose job is to help you understand and effectively navigate the treatment labyrinth. Ask if there's a navigator who could help you and if so, take advantage of it!

- Understanding what is being done to you and why may help you feel more settled and able to focus, in between doctors' appointments, on what matters to you most.

CARPE DIEM

Which question has been bugging you the most today? Take action to try to track down an answer. Notice if the mere act of taking action helps you feel better.

55.

TAKE THINGS ONE DAY AT A TIME

"Life is like an ice-cream cone. You have to lick it one day at a time."
— Charles M. Schulz

- Your grief, like your cancer treatment response, will feel different on different days. Some days will naturally be harder than others.

- Yet each day is a new opportunity—to grieve and mourn, yes, but also to love and to connect.

- When I have a particularly rough day, I sometimes picture a chalkboard covered with all the emotions and conversations and happenings of that day. Then in my imagination, as I lie in bed with my eyes closed, I erase the messy chalkboard. When I'm done erasing, I have a "clean slate" to start with the next morning.

- Take things one day at a time. That's all there is.

CARPE DIEM

Start each new day with a meditation or prayer that helps you live from the heart and be open to all the blessings of that day.

56.

DRINK ENOUGH WATER

"I knew when I was diagnosed with cancer the only thing I could control was what I ate, what I drank, and what I would think."

— Kris Carr

- Our bodies are about 60 percent water, and every system in our bodies depends on water to do its job.

- When you are stressed and focused on your cancer thoughts, feelings, and treatment, you may not feel thirsty. Common cancer treatment side effects, such as vomiting and diarrhea, can also cause dehydration—sometimes severe dehydration.

- How much water you need to drink each day depends on your health and lifestyle. A good rule of thumb is eight cups a day. If your treatment and side effects are making you dehydrated, you'll need to drink even more.

- Carrying a refillable water bottle with you wherever you go is a good habit to start. If you don't like plain water, try adding lemon slices or powdered flavoring. Tea, coffee, and juice count as well, though sugar and caffeine both have dehydrating effects.

- You might not realize that even mild dehydration of one to two percent loss of body weight can sap your energy and make you tired. (One pint of water weighs a pound. So being short just a pint or two is all it takes!) Signs and symptoms of dehydration include excessive thirst, fatigue, headache, dizziness, dry mouth, little urination, and muscle weakness.

- Don't forget to eat foods with high water content as well. Lettuce, watermelon, broccoli, soups, and popsicles all contain lots of water.

CARPE DIEM
If you aren't already in the habit of carrying a water bottle with you wherever you go, buy a refillable container and start today.

57.

FIND BITS OF BEAUTY IN EACH DAY

"I don't think of all the misery but of the beauty that still remains."
— Anne Frank

- One of the most amazing things about life is the Earth's rotation. Because our planet spins, we live each day part in darkness, part in light. And our bodies were built to sleep, to restore, during the period of darkness.

- What this means is that every 24 hours, we live for 16 or so hours then we pause for 8 hours. And after the pause, we awaken to live again.

- It's a cliché, yet every day is indeed a new beginning—but only if you embrace its uniqueness. Each day is a new opportunity for you to connect, to love, to live your truth. And if you screw it up, as we all do, well then, tomorrow's a new day.

- You can't control what happens every day, but you can control how you respond to what happens. In each moment, learn to look for the beauty. Stuck in the wrong grocery line, *again*? Instead of fuming, relax and notice the singular beauty of the face of the person in front of you and silently send her a blessing. In despair over something? Step outside and find something beautiful—a leaf, a bug, a cloud. Spend a few minutes in gratitude for this beauty.

CARPE DIEM

Look around you right now. Pick something beautiful to look at—
something or someone you take for granted but that is actually quite
wonderful. Say a silent prayer of thanks.

58.

TRY VITAMIN C

"Vitamin C is the world's best natural antibiotic, antiviral, antitoxin, and antihistamine. The importance of vitamin C cannot be overemphasized."

— Andrew W. Saul

- The famous biochemist Linus Pauling and a Scottish doctor Ewan Cameron came up with the theory that vitamin C was a key element in the impeding of cancer by strengthening the collagen material that surrounds each cell.

- It is interesting that while most mammals produce vitamin C in their livers, humans are among the few who need to get it from their diet. Vitamin C is an essential vitamin the human body needs to function well. It is a water-soluble vitamin and is found in abundance in citrus fruits such as oranges, grapefruit, and lemons, and in green leafy vegetables, tomatoes, potatoes, strawberries, red and green peppers, and cantaloupe.

- Many scientific studies have shown that diets high in fruits and vegetables (many of which contain vitamin C as well as other vitamins, fiber, and phytochemicals) reduce the risk of cancers of the pancreas, esophagus, larynx, mouth, stomach, colon and rectum, breast, cervix, and lungs.

- The American Cancer Society recommends that adults eat at least two-and-a-half cups of fruits and vegetables every day. Although it is controversial whether vitamin C can actually help to treat cancer, doses under 1,000 milligrams daily are generally thought to be safe. Still, you should check with your cancer care team before you start any supplement.

CARPE DIEM
If you have trouble eating enough fruits and vegetables, consider a vitamin C supplement. But ask your doctor before starting this to be sure it is appropriate with your other treatments.

59.

SPEND TIME IN "THIN PLACES"

"Sacred places are the truest definitions of the earth; they stand for the earth immediately and forever; they are its flags and shields. If you would know the earth for what it really is, learn it through its sacred places. You become one with a spirit that pervades geologic time and space."

— N. Scott Momaday

- In the Celtic tradition, "thin places" are spots where the separation between the physical world and the spiritual world seems tenuous. They are places where the veil between Heaven and earth, between the holy and the everyday, is so thin that when we are near them, we intuitively sense the timeless, boundless spiritual world.

- There is a Celtic saying that heaven and earth are only three feet apart, but in the thin places that distance is even smaller.

- Thin places are usually outdoors, often where water and land meet or land and sky come together. You might find thin places on a riverbank, a beach, or a mountaintop.

- Is there a thin place that is special to you? Go there to feed your spirit.

CARPE DIEM

Your thin places are anywhere that fills you with awe and a sense of wonder. They are spots that refresh your spirit and make you feel closer to God. Go to a thin place today and sit in contemplative silence.

60.

CALM CHRONIC INFLAMMATION

"Chronic inflammation adversely affects survival in many cancers (colon, breast, esophageal, pancreatic, renal cell, head and neck, ovarian, lung, myeloma, and non-Hodgkin's lymphoma) as well as advanced cancer in general."

— D. Barry Boyd and Marian Betancourt

- We now know that chronic, low-grade inflammation in the body may help abnormal cells grow and create conditions for cancer. In fact, inflammation is the engine that drives many of the cancers of middle and old age.

- Many of the attributes of a Western lifestyle, such as a diet high in sugars and saturated fats, along with little or no exercise, make it easy for our bodies to become inflamed…and stay inflamed. Depression, which is common in cancer patients, has also been linked to higher inflammatory cytokines.

- If you aren't already taking optimal care of yourself, your body almost certainly harbors inflammation. You can't see it, but it's there.

- Take steps to reduce inflammation in your body. Lose excess weight, increase exercise, eat less sugar (empty carbs) and animal fat, eat lots of fruits and veggies, choose healthy fats (such as olive oil), nibble on nuts and seeds, and seek treatment if you are experiencing clinical depression. You'll feel better, and you'll be helping your body battle cancer.

CARPE DIEM
Make a list of the ways you can reduce your body's chronic inflammation. Pick one and work on it before moving on to the others.

61.

SAY WHAT YOU NEED TO SAY

"When we were children, we used to think that when we were grown-up we would no longer be vulnerable. But to grow up is to accept vulnerability... To be alive is to be vulnerable."

— Madeleine L'Engle

• Your illness may have you thinking about things you wish you had said or done but never did. These kinds of regrets are normal, and none of us says or does everything that perhaps we should. It's just part of being human.

• While it may be too late to say or do some of these things, it's probably not too late for all of them. Take action while you can.

• Don't wait! None of us ever knows for sure how much precious time on Earth we have left. Don't let another day go by without telling those you love how much they mean to you.

CARPE DIEM

If you're feeling well enough, make a special, individual lunch or dinner date with the most special people in your life—one person at a time. Just the two of you will celebrate your relationship, catch up, and spend an hour or two basking in your love for one another. Over dessert (and yes, there really should be at least a bite or two of dessert for this dinner), take this person's hands in yours and tell him how you feel about him. If your health makes such a meal an impossibility, invite these loved ones to your home, one special meeting at a time.

62.

CONSIDER COMPLEMENTARY THERAPIES

"The greatest mistake in the treatment of diseases is that there are physicians for the body and physicians for the soul, although the two cannot be separated."

— Plato

- The cancer community now knows that the disease and its treatment affect people not just physically and emotionally but also socially, cognitively, and spiritually. That means that treatments targeted to rid the body of cancer cells aren't the only treatments needed.

- You'll be much more comfortable if you seek treatment for the physical side effects, too. Massage, aromatherapy, acupuncture, and yoga are just a few of the complementary therapies (also called integrative therapies) that can help you feel better during and after your course of treatment.

- These same therapies also tend to support your emotions and even your spirituality. Many of them are in essence forms of mourning.

- Also to consider: chiropractic, hypnotherapy, reflexology, healing touch, art therapy, guided imagery, Reiki, pet therapy, music therapy, and various types of herbal and vitamin therapies. (Be sure to talk to your oncologist before you begin eating or drinking anything new.)

CARPE DIEM

Pick a complementary therapy you've been wanting to try but haven't. Learn more about it or make an appointment today.

63.

SIMPLIFY YOUR LIFE

"Our life is frittered away by detail. Simplify, simplify, simplify! I say, let your affairs be as two or three, and not a hundred or a thousand; instead of a million count half a dozen."

— Henry David Thoreau

- Many of us today are taking stock of what's really important in our lives and trying to discard the rest.

- When you are feeling grief about cancer, you are often overwhelmed by all the tasks and commitments you have both in your life and in your treatment. You may be physically ailing. Your body and mind may not be able to function well enough to keep up with your busy schedule. If you can rid yourself of some of those extraneous burdens, you'll have more time for your family and friends and for mourning and healing.

- What is it that is burdening you right now? Have your name taken off junk mail lists, ignore your dirty house, stop attending optional meetings you don't look forward to.

- Ask a friend to help you with running errands, getting groceries, paying bills, etc. Lots of times your friends would like to help but don't know how. This is one practical, tangible way they can.

- If you simplify your life, your mind will be refreshed and more able to handle your life's challenges.

CARPE DIEM

Take at look at your activities calendar. Involve the family. Ask everyone which activities they truly want to continue and which they would be happier without. Make cuts where appropriate. Maybe you can even fill in some of the extra time you'll have with a little vacation.

64.

RELIEVE MUSCLE TENSION
WITH MASSAGE

"When you touch a body, you touch the whole person—the intellect, the spirit, and the emotions."

— Jane Harrington

• Are your neck and shoulders or other parts of your body tight and tense from the stress of dealing with cancer? Consider a soothing massage to relax the muscle tightness and relieve the pain that you feel.

• Maybe you think of massage only as a luxury in exotic spas and upscale health clubs, but did you know that massage therapy, when combined with traditional medical treatments, is used to reduce stress and pain and promote healing in tense muscles? During a massage, a therapist manipulates your body's soft tissues—your muscles, skin, and tendons—using her fingertips, hands, and fists. Several versions of massage are available, and they are performed in a variety of settings.

• Millions of people worldwide turn to massage for relaxation, relief of stress and anxiety, and easing muscle soreness. Massage can also cause your body to release natural painkillers and may boost your immune system.

• Consider an occasional massage as a vital part of the ongoing care and maintenance of your body. Your doctor may be able to refer you to a professional massage therapist, and, in some cases, massage therapy may even be covered by insurance.

• Oncology massage therapists specialize in working with cancer patients to help them relax, sleep better, reduce pain and nausea, and bolster immune function. See if your hospital or clinic offers oncology massage.

CARPE DIEM
Be kind to your body and relieve your stress by scheduling a massage today.

65.

LAUGH

"If you laugh, you think, and you cry, that's a full day. That's a heck of a day. You do that seven days a week, you're going to have something special."

— Jim Valvano

- You've probably heard the story of Norman Cousins, who claimed to have cured himself of a serious illness by watching funny movies. More recently, studies have proven that laughter helps lessen pain, lower stress-related hormones, and boost the immune system, among other benefits.

- Laughter also restores hope and assists us in surviving the pain of grief. If you're of faith, perhaps you'll relate to Proverbs 15:13: "A merry heart is good medicine for the soul."

- No matter your diagnosis or prognosis, it's OK to laugh. In fact, it's good to laugh! Laughter will make both your body and your spirit feel better.

- What has always made you laugh? Whether it's sitcoms, funny movies, comics in the newspaper, or certain friends, try to schedule some laugh time into each and every day.

CARPE DIEM

What can you do today that is sure to tickle your funny bone and take your mind off your troubles, if only for a few minutes? Do it.

66.

CRY

"Sometimes allowing yourself to cry is the scariest thing you'll ever do. And the bravest. It takes a lot of courage to face the facts, stare loss in the face, bare your heart, and let it bleed. But it is the only way to cleanse your wounds and prepare them for healing."

— Barbara Johnson

- Tears are a natural cleansing and healing mechanism. It's OK to cry. In fact, it's good to cry when you feel like it. What's more, tears are a form of mourning. They are sacred!

- On the other hand, don't feel bad if you aren't crying a lot. Not everyone is a crier. Some men, in particular, do not feel the need to cry. The inability to cry is not necessarily a deficit.

- You may find that those around you are uncomfortable with your tears. As a society, we're often not so good at witnessing others in pain.

- Explain to your friends and family that you need to cry right now and that they can help by allowing you to.

- You may find yourself crying at unexpected times or places. If you need to, excuse yourself and retreat to somewhere private.

CARPE DIEM

If you feel like it, have a good cry today. Find a safe place to embrace your pain and cry as long and as hard as you want to.

67.

TAKE A FIVE-MINUTE SPIRIT BREAK

"Nobody sees a flower really; it is so small. We haven't time, and to see takes time—like to have a friend takes time."

— Georgia O'Keefe

- Sometimes it may feel like the experience of cancer has thoroughly drained your spirit and sucked out your soul.

- In these moments, when you feel dead or in despair or ready to give up, make an effort to connect with your spirituality.

- Set everything aside and take five minutes for a spiritual practice of your choosing.

- What can you do in five minutes? You can meditate. You can pray. You can do a yoga pose or two. You can journal your gratitude. You can take a walk through a park. You can listen to music that fills you with hope and joy. You can hold someone you love. You can close your eyes and visualize heaven.

CARPE DIEM

Stop what you are doing and take a five-minute spirit break. Set the timer on your oven or on your phone. You might be surprised by how refreshed you can feel in just five minutes.

68.

CULTIVATE RESILIENCE

"Once I overcame breast cancer, I wasn't afraid of anything anymore."
— Melissa Etheridge

• Resilience is the character trait that encourages you to get back up after you've been knocked down.

• We would also like to emphasize, however, that resilience does NOT mean pretending that nothing bad is happening or denying that it hurt to get knocked down. Absolutely not! In fact, the whole point of this book is insisting that you acknowledge and express the many hurts of cancer.

• BUT (and this is a big but) you can, over time, use your cancer as a springboard to resilience. After all…you've already experienced one of the most difficult struggles in life. Doesn't that give you a new perspective on whatever else might come your way?

• We all know certain people who've been through a lot and yet still seem energetic and joyful about life. Maybe you could make it a point to talk to a couple of these survivor types about how they cultivate resilience.

CARPE DIEM
Read an inspiring true book about someone who championed over hardship.

69.

WRITE LETTERS TO BE READ ON A FUTURE DATE

"How wonderful it is to be able to write someone a letter! To feel like conveying your thoughts to a person, to sit at your desk and pick up a pen, to put your thoughts into words like this is truly marvelous."
— Haruki Murakami

- No matter your prognosis, your cancer probably has you thinking about what will happen after you're gone—whether that's five weeks from now or five decades. It's hard but natural to consider what your partner, your friends, your children, or your grandchildren would remember about you or how their lives would be affected by your absence.

- There is a way for you talk to your loved ones after you're gone—and no, we're not talking about supernatural communication. You can write them letters now to be opened upon your death or at specified times in the future.

- Let's say your first grandchild will soon be born. What might you say to her on her 18th birthday? Maybe you'll have the good fortune to attend her 18th birthday party, but in case you won't, you can take the opportunity now to share, with love and in writing, all the heartfelt wisdom and good wishes you would shower on her in person. (And since they'll be in the form of a letter, she might even read and listen to them!)

CARPE DIEM

Buy some nice stationery and write a letter today to be opened either upon your death or on a certain, specified date. Give the letter to your attorney or someone who will safeguard it for you yet not forget it exists.

70.

TAP INTO YOUR INTUITION

"The intuitive mind is a sacred gift, and the rational mind is a faithful servant. We have created a society that honors the servant and has forgotten the gift."

— Albert Einstein

- Few psychologists would deny that we possess a subtle, intuitive part of our mind that can be a great source of strength, joy, and creative insight. Steve Jobs, in his famous Stanford University commencement address, advised students not to let the "noise of others' opinions drown out your own inner voice," but rather "have the courage to follow your heart and intuition." Wise advice for us all.

- Although throughout your cancer journey it is important to listen to the information you get from experts, it's also important in your treatment and recovery for you to listen to your intuitive mind. You often know best what is the right thing for you in facing your cancer, maximizing your immune system's response, and allowing yourself to find your own path to recovery.

- Think of your intuition as one tool in your cancer-fighting toolkit. If you have a strong "gut feeling" that you should or should not do something that has been suggested to you, consider going with your gut. After all, much of cancer treatment is still an imprecise science, and intuition is sometimes our best decision-making tool.

CARPE DIEM

Meditate, or try other methods of clearing your mind, such as stretching, yoga, or deep breathing. After these mind-clearing exercises, listen to what first comes into your mind when you again face your problems. Now rationally look at this intuitive thought. Does it make sense? Do you believe it?

71.

GET ENOUGH VITAMIN D

"Something so simple—vitamin D supplementation—could improve the health status of millions and so becomes an elegant solution to many of our health problems today."

— Carol L Wagner, MD

- Researchers have found that vitamin D deficiency is an important factor in the development of cancer as well as autoimmune disorders like rheumatoid arthritis, lupus, and multiple sclerosis.

- Due to the combination of low sun exposure and lack of vitamin D in the diet, about 70 percent of adults in the U.S. are deficient in this vital vitamin. Worldwide, it's estimated that about one billion people don't get enough vitamin D. The good news is that a simple lab test can check your vitamin D levels.

- Oily fish like salmon, mackerel, and tuna are good sources of vitamin D. Egg yolks and mushrooms are also rich in vitamin D. Some people rely on vitamin D-fortified milk or cereals as their source. Your body also makes its own vitamin D from sunlight, but it is not recommended to spend too much in the sun without sunscreen.

- Vitamin D helps with the absorption of calcium and preventing osteoporosis. It also wards off mood problems like depression, and may even help ease musculoskeletal pain and optimize our immune systems.

- Optimize your body's function by optimizing your vitamin D level, and take advantage of its cancer-fighting properties.

CARPE DIEM

Make an appointment with your doctor and discuss checking your vitamin D with a specialized test called a 25-hydroxy vitamin D level. It's just a simple blood draw, but it can give you and your doctor important information.

72.

DRINK FRESH-SQUEEZED JUICE

"It's possible to forget how alive we really are. We can become dry and tired, just existing, instead of really living. We need to remind ourselves of the juice of life, and make that a habit. Find those places inside that jump for joy...and do things."

— Author unknown

- Everybody knows that fruits and veggies are chockfull of vitamins and antioxidants—nutrition that can help jumpstart your body's immune system and help it fight off cancer. But you can only eat so many of them in a day, right?

- Juicing is a way to squeeze way more of the nutritious benefits of fruits and vegetables into your diet. Juices also help keep you hydrated.

- Dr. Oz's famous "Green Drink," which he reportedly has for breakfast every morning, contains two apples, three stalks of celery, half a cucumber, one-quarter of a lemon, one-quarter of a lime, half a bunch of parsley, one bunch of mint, three carrots, one-quarter of a pineapple, and two cups of spinach. Throw it all into a blender, blend well, and drink up.

- Don't forget to wash your fruit before juicing. And if you're not up to juicing at home, you can buy freshly squeezed juices at natural grocery stores and juice bars.

- Think of it this way: Juices and other healthy foods will give you fuel to do the things that matter most to you in the coming weeks and months—including mourning.

CARPE DIEM
Today, learn about juicing from someone who does it regularly. Try out a simple juice recipe at home and see what you think.

73.

DON'T BE ALARMED BY "GRIEFBURSTS"

"In the first few months of my grief, nothing could distract me from the sorrow and pain. When you quit trying to avoid the breakdowns, the grief bursts, the weeping episodes, you feel better. I don't think you can force yourself to stop. People try, but it's ultimately what keeps them from healing."

— Bruce Lee

- Sometimes heightened periods of sadness overwhelm us when we're in grief. These moments can seem to come out of nowhere and can be frightening and painful.

- Even long after your diagnosis and treatment, something as simple as a sound, a smell, or a phrase can bring on a "griefburst." You might hear a name, see a building, or feel a twinge that suddenly reminds you of your cancer and all you have gone through.

- Allow yourself to experience griefbursts without shame or self-judgment, no matter where and when they occur. (Sooner or later, one will probably happen when you're surrounded by people, maybe even strangers.) If you would feel more comfortable, retreat to somewhere private when these strong feelings surface.

- Don't isolate yourself in an attempt to protect yourself from griefbursts, however. Staying cooped up at home all the time is not self-compassion: it's self-destruction.

CARPE DIEM
Create an action plan for your next griefburst. For example, you might plan to drop whatever you are doing and go for a walk or record thoughts in your journal.

74.

LIVE IN THE NOW

"What day is it?"
"It's today," squeaked Piglet.
"My favorite day," said Pooh.

— A.A. Milne

- You may have heard it said that there is no past, there is no future, there is only this moment.

- In his bestselling book *The Power of Now*, Eckhart Tolle encourages us to truly be present in the current moment. "Life is now," he writes. "There was never a time when your life was not now, nor will there ever be… Nothing ever happened in the past; it happened in the Now. Nothing will ever happen in the future; it will happen in the Now."

- The challenge is that it is really *hard* to live in the moment. Our minds constantly revisit the past and think forward to the future. Our egos dwell on what was and what will be. Especially when we are uncertain about our futures, we tend to obsess about what *could* happen. Uncertainty makes us anxious.

- The next time you find yourself ruminating about what *might* happen, consciously pull yourself to the present moment. Look— really look—at your surroundings. Take a deep breath and discern what you smell. Reach out to touch several different textures within arm's reach. Listen to the sounds you hear. Consider the power of Now and revel in this moment.

CARPE DIEM

Right now, empty your mind of its concerns and just "be" in this moment. Breathe in; breathe out. Find at least one thing around you to marvel about or give thanks for.

75.

SEEK OUT A SPIRITUAL ADVISOR

"If you want to go fast, go alone; if you want to go far, go with others."
— African proverb

- Many of us flounder in our spirituality, especially in the early weeks and months after a cancer diagnosis.

- To assist you in your search for meaning and to provide you with spiritual mentoring, seek out the help of someone whom you find to be spiritually advanced or grounded.

- This person might be a member of the clergy or someone with formal religious or spiritual training, but it also might be someone who simply seems to connect well with the spiritual realm.

- You also might find it helpful to seek the spiritual advice of a fellow cancer survivor or someone who has experienced significant life challenges.

CARPE DIEM
Right now, make a list of three local people you look up to spiritually. Try to identify someone with whom you can meet in person periodically. Call him or her today and extend an invitation to meet for coffee.

76.

MEND FENCES

"But grief makes a monster out of us sometimes…and sometimes you say and do things to the people you love that you can't forgive yourself for."

— Melina Marchetta

- If old hurts or transgressions are hindering any significant relationships in your life, now may be the time to mend fences.

- One of the six needs of mourning is receiving (and accepting) help from others. But if "bad blood" is separating you from some of them, how can you be there for each other?

- We can't change other people, but we can change our own behavior. And sometimes when we say "I'm sorry" (even if what happened wasn't clearly our fault), we open a closed door just enough to let love flow through again.

- Yes, sometimes it's better to set boundaries so that toxic people can't enter at all. But often, we can rebuild relationships with even "difficult" people by simply extending an olive branch and approaching with kindness.

CARPE DIEM

What one relationship in your life is the most strained? Is it a source of pain for you? If so, the pain is a sign that you should express your thoughts and feelings. Find someone else who's a good listener and unburden yourself today. Consider next steps.

77.

SIGH

"You will find that it is necessary to let things go, simply for the reason that they are heavy. So let them go, let go of them. I tie no weights to my ankles."

— C. Joy Bell

- Sighing is an expression of letting go. When we sigh, we resign ourselves to something. We accept something, though perhaps it is something we didn't want to accept. It helps release the tension in our bodies.

- In Romans 8 it says that when there are no words for our prayer, the spirits intervene and pray for us in sighs deeper than anything that can be expressed in words.

- Sigh deeply. Sigh whenever you feel like it. With each sigh, you are acknowledging that you are not in total control of your life. You are accepting what is. Accepting your cancer, your treatment…and your life.

- Each sigh is your prayer.

CARPE DIEM
Right now, take a deep breath and sigh. Do this ten times in a row.
How do you feel?

78.

BEWARE THE NOCEBO EFFECT

"Beliefs have the power to create and the power to destroy. Human beings have the awesome ability to take any experience of their lives and create a meaning that disempowers them or one that can literally save their lives."

— Anthony Robbins

- Have you heard of the nocebo effect? It's the placebo effect's evil twin.

- As you know, the placebo effect is the improvement of symptoms or outcomes based simply on belief. If a doctor gives you a sugar pill but tells you that it is medicine that will make you better, you are, in fact, more likely to get better than others who didn't receive the placebo pill.

- The nocebo effect is the opposite. People who are warned about pain or side effects before a treatment are, studies prove, more likely to report pain or side effects afterward.

- The mind is a powerful creator. Thoughts can indeed create, or at least foster, reality.

- While it's natural to be afraid and to consider the worst after a cancer diagnosis or follow-up testing, keep in mind the nocebo effect. If we convince ourselves that cancer will kill us, there is evidence to suggest that we could be tipping the scales in cancer's favor.

CARPE DIEM

If dark, pessimistic thoughts seem to be consuming you, consider talking to a counselor trained in Cognitive Behavioral Therapy. A CBT therapist can give you tools to adjust your thought patterns. Meditation can also help you clear your mind and focus instead on a positive mantra.

79.

CELEBRATE WORLD CANCER DAY

"If you are utterly close to someone battling cancer, there is one sure thing you can say to make them feel even a shred of a whiff of a modicum of better: "I will be here for you in any way you need, in any way I can."

— Dan Duffy

- World Cancer Day is the first Tuesday in February.
- What if everybody spent that one day each year doing something to prevent or find a cure for or help someone with cancer? We wonder how many more World Cancer Days there would have to be...
- Consider spending the day honoring and remembering your cancer journey in some way. Maybe you want to do something special with your family or partner.
- You could also mark the day by donating to cancer research or signing up to be a volunteer at your local hospital or hospice. Or, perhaps you know someone else living with cancer. What if you spent the day being a compassionate companion to this person?

CARPE DIEM
Mark the next World Cancer Day on your calendar and plan something special.

80.

BE MINDFUL OF ANNIVERSARIES

"Yesterday was the three-year anniversary of my diagnosis. It is weird the way I will start to get stressed when it gets close to that date, even still. Yesterday, though, I bought a bottle of champagne and celebrated still being alive."

— A posting on Cancer Survivors Network

- Throughout your cancer journey, anniversaries of all kinds—of the day you found a lump, of the day of your diagnosis, of the day you finished radiation or chemotherapy, of your birthday or wedding anniversary, of the day a friend or family member died—may be difficult.

- These are times you may want to plan ahead for. Consider what would be a meaningful way for you to spend the next anniversary that's approaching.

- Others, even those closest to you, may not remember the exact date of your diagnosis or last chemo treatment. Don't expect them to, and try not to feel hurt when they don't.

- Instead, reach out. If you want to spend the day connecting with those you love, be proactive in letting them know. Call up your best friend and say, "Next Tuesday is the anniversary of my surgery. I was hoping we could have dinner."

- On the other hand, if you feel like turning inward on the next anniversary, that's OK too. All of us need times of contemplative silence and spiritual reflection. Consider spending the day in a place that feeds your soul and allows you to embrace your spirituality.

CARPE DIEM

What's the next anniversary you've been anticipating? Make a plan right now for what you will do on that day.

81.

PLANT A TREE

"I'm planting a tree to teach me to gather strength from my deepest roots."

— Andrea Koehle Jones

- Gardening is not only good exercise—it's good for the heart and soul. If you're a gardener, try to find ways to keep your hands in the dirt at least a little during your cancer journey. (But do wear gloves to protect yourself from germs.)

- But even if you're not a gardener, you can plant a tree. Your tree will serve as a reminder of a positive action you chose to take during your illness. Season after season, you can watch it grow bigger and stronger.

- If you choose a deciduous tree, you can watch it leaf out in the spring, maybe blossom with flowers, create a lovely canopy of shade, and then change color in the fall and drop its leaves. It's the circle of life, right out your window. Watching and tending your new tree can be a way of touching base with your cancer feelings, which will change and wither and reemerge much in the way the tree does.

- Of course, planting a tree is, at bottom, a metaphor for creating something that will live on long after you're gone. No matter how many more decades you live here on Earth, it's your children and grandchildren who will most benefit from the trees you plant. If you don't want to or can't plant an actual tree, what can you do instead to create something that will help your friends and family always remember you?

CARPE DIEM
Consider where you could plant a tree and make plans to do it.

82.

PRAY

"On the day I called, you answered me; my strength of soul you increased."

— Psalms 138:3

- Prayer is mourning because prayer means taking your feelings and articulating them to someone else. Even when you pray silently, you're forming words for your thoughts and feelings and you're offering up those words to a presence outside yourself.
- Someone wise once noted, "Our faith is capable of reaching the realm of mystery."
- Did you know that real medical studies have shown that prayer can actually help people heal?
- If you believe in a higher power, pray. Pray for your own health. Pray for others affected by your cancer. Pray for your questions about life and death to be answered. Pray for the strength to persevere in your journey through cancer and to find continued meaning in life and living.
- Many places of worship have prayer lists. Call yours and ask that your name be added to the prayer list. On worship days, the whole congregation will pray for you. Often many individuals will pray at home for those on the prayer list, as well.

CARPE DIEM
Bow your head right now and say a silent prayer. If you are out of practice, don't worry; just let your thoughts flow naturally.

83.

MAKE TIME FOR MUSIC

"Some days there won't be a song in your heart. Sing anyway."
— Emory Austin

- We've noticed that music is something it's easy to stop making time for. Most people love music when they are children and teenagers. But in our busy adult lives, we sometimes let go of it.

- If you once loved music but haven't listened much lately, now's a good time to fire up the old record player again (or iPod, Pandora, etc.). Music will help you feel your feelings. It's also really good at soothing you when you're feeling anxious and lifting you up when you're feeling down.

- Basically, music is a mood massager.

- Feeling nostalgic? Play music from your teenage years. Need a good cry? Listen to some Sarah McLachlan or Josh Groban. Tired of crying and feeling blue? Pick out something upbeat and dancey.

CARPE DIEM
Try taking a short walk today while listening to music through headphones. Music and movement *together* combine to help you in so many ways.

84.

REASSESS YOUR PRIORITIES

*"The life you have left is a gift. Cherish it. Enjoy it now, to the fullest.
Do what matters, now."*

— Leo Babauta

• Cancer has a way of making us rethink our lives and the
meaningfulness of the ways we spend them.

• What gives your life meaning? What doesn't? Take steps to spend
more of your time on the former and less on the latter.

• Now may be the time to reconfigure your life. Choose a satisfying
new second career or hobby. Go back to school. Begin volunteering.
Help others in regular, ongoing ways. Move closer to your children
and grandchildren.

• Many people living with cancer have told me that they can no longer
stand to be around people who seem shallow, egocentric, or mean-
spirited. It's OK to let friendships wither with friends whom these
adjectives now seem to describe. Instead, find ways to connect with
people who share your new outlook on life—and death.

CARPE DIEM
Make a list with two columns: What's important to me. What's not.
Brainstorm for at least 15 minutes.

85.

WEAR PRAYER BEADS

"I thought that I had no time for faith nor time to pray, then I saw an armless man saying his rosary with his feet."

— John Locke

- People in many spiritual traditions wear prayer beads. You'll find them around the necks of Christians, Hindus, Buddhists, Sikhs, Muslims, and others.

- Did you know that the word "bead" comes from the Old English term *bede*, which means prayer?

- Prayer beads are strings of beads, often made of wood, and are composed of certain numbers and patterns characteristic of their respective faith traditions. Buddhists and Hindus wear "malas," which are comprised of 108 beads (four sets of 27). Roman Catholics wear rosaries, which have 54 beads plus five hanging down from the center, ending in a cross.

- Regardless of your specific beliefs, you can wear prayer beads to help center you whenever you are feeling anxious or ruminating on negative thoughts. (Prayer beads are also called "worry beads"!) Take them from around your neck and hold them in your hands. Finger the beads. Say an affirmation for each bead you touch: "I am resilient." (move to the next bead) "I am hopeful." (move to the next bead) "I am loved."

CARPE DIEM
Visit a spiritual or religious shop in your community today and pick out a string of prayer beads.

86.

WATCH FOR WARNING SIGNS

"Accept everything about yourself—I mean everything. You are you and that is the beginning and the end—no apologies, no regrets."

— Clark Moustakas

- Understandably, sometimes people with cancer are so stressed that they fall back on self-destructive behaviors to get through this difficult time.

- Try to be honest with yourself about drug or alcohol abuse. If you're in over your head, ask someone for help. If others approach you about your substance abuse, let them in.

- Of course, mental illness and personality problems that were present before your diagnosis can also complicate your cancer grief.

- Seeing a grief counselor is probably a good idea for people with cancer who are also struggling with substance abuse, clinical depression, or other mental health-related problems. You may simply not be able to reconcile your grief and continue your life in a meaningful way without professional help.

- Are you seriously considering suicide? Put this book down right now and talk to someone about your depression. Get the help you need and deserve immediately!

CARPE DIEM
Acknowledging to ourselves that we have a problem may come too late. If someone suggests that you need help, consider yourself lucky to be so well loved and get help.

87.

GO EASY ON PEOPLE WHO SAY STUPID THINGS

"Two things are infinite: the universe and human stupidity; and I'm not sure about the universe."

— Albert Einstein

- I'm sure you've realized by now that people don't know what to say to someone who has cancer. Often they say the wrong things:
    - "It will be OK. I just know it."
    - "Don't do chemo! It's better to _____."
    - "Everything happens for a reason."
    - "Lance Armstrong cured his Stage IV cancer."
    - "Someday you'll look back on this and be grateful."
    - "Cancer means you're repressing anger or negative emotions."
    - "You'll grow so much stronger because of this."
    - "All you need to do is think positive."
    - "Be strong. Keep your chin up."
- When I was diagnosed, someone said, "Just think etc. now you can write a really good book about cancer." Of course, that was the last thing I wanted to do early on. But, down the line, writing this book has helped me in my search for meaning. Have grace.
- Most of these people are well intentioned. They truly don't realize how phrases like these diminish your unique loss. As Maya Angelou wrote, "You did what you knew how to do, and when you knew better, you did better."
- Sometimes entering into an honest, deeper discussion with such people about what cancer has really been like for you is a way to break through the clichés, helping them as well as you.

CARPE DIEM

Try talking with your partner (or a close friend) about the hurtful remarks others sometimes make. Say, "Aren't you disappointed when people say…?" This conversation may help you express your feelings of hurt and frustration.

88.

CLEAR THE CLUTTER

"Clutter is not just physical stuff. It's old ideas, toxic relationships, and bad habits. Clutter is anything that does not support your better self."
— Eleanor Brown

• Cancer = a lot going on. It's hectic and chaotic, especially in the early days and weeks of diagnosis and treatment. Making your home a serene oasis will help soothe you and unburden your already overburdened mind and soul. Studies even prove that when your environment is cluttered, you're more likely to feel distracted and irritable.

• Ask a good friend or an organized family member to help you clear the clutter in your home.

• Start with the room you spend the most time in. First, clear off all the flat surfaces completely. Pick up stray belongings off the floor and eliminate visual clutter from tabletops, countertops, shelves. Try clearing *all* of it away for now—every last bit. Donate what you don't really love anymore, give away a few keepsakes to people who will appreciate them, and box up the rest.

• Designate an attractive basket for mail and another one for prescriptions.

• Displaying photos of loved ones can help give you strength, but it can also create clutter. Could some of the frames be hung in a nice arrangement on the wall, instead?

• Now place a small, simple arrangement of freshly cut flowers on a table where you'll see it often.

CARPE DIEM
Ask someone to help you de-clutter one room (or part of one room) today.

89.

MAKE A "BAD NEWS" PLAN

"The world is round, and the place which may seem like the end may also be only the beginning."

— Ivy Baker Priest

- It's the uncertainty of cancer that gets us. None of us likes living in limbo. As human beings, we're wired to require a sense of safety and security. (See Idea 6.)

- Specifically, what we don't like about uncertainty is that something bad could happen. In cancer, we talk about stages and odds and percentages—all numbers that try to quantify the possibility of negative developments. Even those of us who were fortunate to receive a good initial prognosis struggle with the "what ifs" and the "worst-case scenarios."

- So what if you do receive bad or worse news during your cancer journey? What will you do? Having a "bad news" plan may help you rest a little easier during your time of limbo.

- Like an emergency preparedness plan, your bad news plan might even be written down. Where will you go? Who will you call? Consider telling a good friend about your plan: "If something bad comes up, I'm going to call you, OK? I'm going to ask you to drop whatever you're doing and come hang out with me so I can talk about it." If you work outside the home, consider telling your boss the same thing: "If I disappear one day for a while, it's probably because I just received bad medical news. I'll be in touch as soon as I can."

CARPE DIEM

In your journal, make some notes about your bad news plan and give the people involved a heads-up.

90.

WRANGLE WORRY

"If a problem is fixable, if a situation is such that you can do something about it, then there is no need to worry. If it's not fixable, then there is no help in worrying. There is no benefit in worrying whatsoever."
— Dalai Lama XIV

- Whether or not you're a natural worrywart may have something to do with your upbringing. People who come from divorced homes are more likely to have generalized anxiety disorder, which means they are chronic worriers. Overprotective parents can create worrier children as well.

- People with cancer tend to worry a lot. We worry about what will happen—if our cancer will go into remission, if it will return, how we will pay for treatment, what will happen to our families if we die—and on and on and on. The worries are endless. And understandable.

- We've said that feelings aren't right or wrong, they just are. This is true of worry too. Learning to express worry every time you're feeling it is the ticket. Here are some techniques to try:

  -Make a written list of your worries.
  -Look over the list and decide which worries you can do something about—and then do it.
  -If you're worried about who would take care of your children if you couldn't, for example, have a heart-to-heart with the person whom you would like to serve as guardian.
  -Practice living in the now (see Idea 74).
  -Talk to several different people about your biggest worries.
  -See a grief counselor.
  -Cry, scream, punch a punching bag.

CARPE DIEM

What is your biggest worry right now? Can you do something about it? If you can, take steps today to begin to put that worry to rest. If you can't, talk to someone about it.

91.

CATCH THE BOUNCE

"A man who carries a cat by the tail learns something he can learn in no other way."

— Mark Twain

- At some point in your cancer journey, you'll probably feel like you're plummeting down, down, down. First the diagnosis and then surgery and/or chemotherapy and/or radiation. It often gets worse and then worse again.

- You finally hit rock bottom, and then what? And then you bounce.

- Bouncing back from cancer isn't fast or easy. It's more of a slow-motion bounce. But if you visualize yourself hitting bottom, balling yourself up as you absorb the pain of impact, you can then ride the energy of that impact up and out.

- Depending on your prognosis, you may have several bounces along the way.

- So, feel the pain of impact and express it. Use the energy you may feel after a time of restoration and contemplation to go further, be braver, open yourself to more joy than you ever have before.

CARPE DIEM
Make a list of things you want to do or say or try the next time you're having a bounce day.

92.

LIVE WITH GRATITUDE AND COUNT YOUR BLESSINGS

"Gratitude unlocks the fullness of life. It turns what we have into enough, and more. It turns denial into acceptance, chaos to order, confusion to clarity. It can turn a meal into a feast, a house into a home, a stranger into a friend."

— Melody Beattie

- When you are faced with a horrible disease like cancer, and you feel the pain and the losses, it can be difficult to have a sense of gratitude about your life, yet gratitude prepares you for the blessings yet to come.

- Many blessings have already been companioning you since you started on this cancer journey. Somehow, and with grace, you have survived. Think back and recognize the many supportive gestures, big and small, you have already been offered along the way.

- When you fill your life with gratitude, you invoke a self-fulfilling prophecy. What you expect to happen *can* happen. If you anticipate support and nurturance, you will find it. If you don't expect anyone to support you, often they don't.

- Think of all that you have to be thankful for. This is not to minimize the difficulty of your present situation but to allow you to reflect on the possibilities for love and joy each day. Honor those possibilities and have gratitude for them. Be grateful for your life and strong spirit. Be grateful for your family and friends and the time you can still share. Above all, be grateful for this very moment. When you are grateful, you prepare the way for inner peace.

CARPE DIEM

Start keeping a gratitude journal or adding a note of gratitude to each entry in your regular journal. Each night before bed, record the blessings from the day. At first this may seem challenging, but if you continue the daily practice, it will get easier and more joyful.

93.

HAMMER OUT YOUR HOPES

"Once you choose hope, anything's possible."
— Christopher Reeve

• Hope is an expectation of a good that is yet to be. No matter what your prognosis is, you can have hope for good things—big or small—that may yet happen.

• Hope is a bit different from optimism, which is a general feeling that good things will happen. Hope comes from having goals and dreams together with the desire and plans to reach them.

• What do you hope for? Now what can you do to work toward achieving those hopes?

• You have a powerful and amazing life force. You can make things happen. You can ask for help. You can seek advice. You can do one small thing each day to move closer to your hopes. You can trust that everything will be OK.

• If you are not a naturally hopeful person, try talking to someone who is. Ask them how they might think about your cancer journey if they were in your shoes.

CARPE DIEM

Today, talk to someone else about what you hope for. Don't forget to tell that person what you plan to do to make those hopes a reality.

94.

MAKE GOALS AND PLANS THAT HAVE NOTHING TO DO WITH CANCER

"Be a dreamer. If you don't know how to dream, you're dead."

— Jim Valvano

- Cancer puts your life on hold. Like a tantrum-prone toddler, it can demand all your time and energy for months (and sometimes years) on end.

- But after you've grown used to the rhythms of cancer treatment and doctors' appointments, you might realize that you're ready to start thinking again about plans for *after* cancer.

- When you make goals or plans that extend beyond your cancer treatment window, you're giving yourself something to look forward to. You're cultivating hope. You're also visualizing a future in which you are finding meaning and having fun.

- You can (and should, when you feel up to it) also make goals and plans that have nothing to do with cancer—even while you're still receiving treatment. These are the little perks and joys that can keep you going. Activities like having coffee with a friend or splurges like getting a manicure will brighten your days and help you remember that there is goodness and joy, even during cancer.

CARPE DIEM
Set a goal or make a plan for six months from now. Put it on your calendar.

95.

GIVE YOURSELF UP TO GRIEF

"Something amazing happens when we surrender and just love. We melt into another world, a realm of power already within us. The world changes when we change. The world softens when we soften. The world loves us when we choose to love the world."

— Marianne Williamson

- One of the most common words associated with cancer is "fight." Another is "battle." I understand the urge, the need, to fight for your life. It's built into us—the instinct to fight or flee. And since there is no fleeing from cancer, the only choice we have is to fight it.

- When it comes to grief, however, I have learned that no good comes of fighting it. When we try to deny it, suppress it, shake it off, or keep our chins up, we are not being honest. And when we are not honest with ourselves and with those who care about us, we only compound our pain and distance ourselves from what is good and true.

- Life and death are largely mysteries. We can never understand why some people get sick, why some die too soon. Instead of fighting to understand, we can learn to "stand under" the mystery.

- And when it comes to cancer itself, acceptance is not the same thing as quitting. You can accept your life each day as it is—even as, from a longer standpoint, you continue to fight your cancer.

- If and under what circumstances you might choose to stop fighting for your life is a very personal and individual decision. But even if you never have to or choose to relinquish yourself to cancer, you must relinquish yourself to your grief. Even if you are fighting for your life, you can and must submit to your most honest thoughts and feelings. Give yourself up to them, express them, and be healed.

CARPE DIEM

Write this on a sticky note and place it somewhere you'll see it often: I surrender to my feelings of loss. I surrender to my truest thoughts and feelings. I surrender to the need to receive and accept help from others.

96.

BEWARE THE SNAKE OIL SALESMAN

"Learn from yesterday, live for today, hope for tomorrow. The important thing is not to stop questioning."

— Albert Einstein

- Cancer can make us vulnerable. We're scared, and sometimes we're desperate. This desperation may make us vulnerable to people and companies promising miracle cures and false hopes.
- You know what they say: If something sounds too good to be true, it probably is.
- BUT, and this is a big but, it's also true that the mere act of believing in something can make the desired outcome more likely. What's more, modern medicine doesn't have it all figured out when it comes to cancer. So, sometimes taking a leap of faith is the best way to foster hope.
- If you're trying an unorthodox treatment or therapy, be sure to let your care team know. Certain remedies and protocols might interfere with those that they've prescribed.
- When it comes to grief, the snake oil salesman is the person who insists that you need to forget your troubles and trust that everything will be fine. Or that a pill will make everything better. Not only will denying or medicating your cancer grief not heal you, it will probably make your cancer journey more painful over the long haul.

CARPE DIEM
Who's the most sensible yet open-minded person you know? If you're considering going off the standard cancer treatment rails, talk to this person first.

97.

IF YOUR CANCER IS RECURRING, CHRONIC, OR TERMINAL

"When the time comes to die, make sure that all you have to do is die."
— Jim Elliot

- If your cancer is recurring, chronic, or has been deemed terminal, your cancer grief journey will be especially hard.

- The six needs of mourning (Ideas 8 to 13) apply a hundredfold to you. Please spend some extra time considering them and contemplating how you can continue to meet those needs.

- Cancer changes your life. Chronic cancer can take your life around a sharp corner and onto a totally different path than you ever imagined traveling. Terminal cancer brings you face-to-face with your life's end.

- If you know you are dying, you have been presented with an exceedingly difficult and contradictory challenge: you are dying, you know you are dying, yet it is your nature to want to live. We do not pretend to fully understand what you are going through, but we do understand it as a kind of grief journey.

- In these circumstances, we encourage you to make grief therapy part of your care. A skilled and compassionate professional grief companion can help you not just survive your final days but live and love as fully as possible.

CARPE DIEM
Ask your care team's social worker or a hospice caregiver for a referral to a local grief counselor.

98.

UNWRAP THE GIFTS OF CANCER

"Breast cancer changes you, and the change can be beautiful."
— Jane Cook

- OK, here's where we talk about the "gifts of cancer." Early in our cancer journeys, it's annoying and sometimes downright hurtful when others insist that cancer is a gift.

- "My cancer made me realize what life is all about!" they say. "If it weren't for cancer, I wouldn't be so close to my friends and family… I would still be wasting my time doing… I would never have had the courage to…" They practically glow with the "salvation" of cancer.

- In the beginning, and maybe forever, we despise cancer. We wish it had never grown inside us. We would trade all our material wealth to never have had it. So when people tell us that cancer is a gift, of course we're angry! They're belittling our hurt and despair *before we've had a chance to embrace those feelings and come to terms with them!*

- But we also know, from our own experience as well as from companioning others through cancer, that over time and with the support of others, to mourn our cancer fully and honestly is to not only heal…it's to grow. We *do* change through cancer—often for the better. Our lives *do* often become richer and more meaningful.

- So when you're ready…yes, do unwrap the gifts of cancer. But first you must mourn your way through the pain and the sadness and the anger and the guilt and the helplessness and all those other hurtful thoughts and feelings.

CARPE DIEM
If and only if you're ready to unwrap the gifts of cancer, tell someone else about one of these gifts today. (If you're not ready, completely skip this idea for now!)

99.

UNDERSTAND THAT YOUR GRIEF WILL NEVER END

"Once cancer happens, it changes the way you live for the rest of your life."
— Hayley Mills

- Your cancer grief will never completely go away. Even if you recover completely from your cancer (and we hope you do) and are cancer-free decades from now, you will never truly "recover" from the losses of cancer.

- No, you do not "get over" grief. Even if you are a cancer survivor, you are not the same person after cancer as you were before cancer. You cannot make the memories of your cancer go away. Neither can those who love you. You are unalterably changed, as are they. This happens after all significant loss experiences in life.

- If you mourn well, however—if you fully express your thoughts and feelings of loss and work through your grief—you will reconcile yourself to your cancer and grief experience.

- You will find that as you achieve reconciliation, the sharp, ever-present pain of your cancer grief will give rise to a renewed sense of meaning and purpose. Your feeling of loss will not completely disappear, yet they will soften, and the intense pangs of grief will become less frequent. Hope for a continued life will re-emerge as you are able to make commitments to the future. The unfolding of this journey is not intended to create a return to an "old normal" but instead the discovery of a "new normal."

CARPE DIEM

Think about other significant losses in your life. Have you "gotten over" the death of a parent or a child or a good friend? No. But how has your grief changed over time?

100.

BELIEVE IN YOUR CAPACITY TO HEAL AND GROW THROUGH GRIEF

"Don't go through life. Grow through life."

— Eric Butterworth

- In time, you may find that you are growing emotionally and spiritually as a result of your cancer grief journey. As we said in Idea 98, you may not be ready to discuss growth yet. But even if you're not ready, you can still believe that it's out there waiting for you.

- Growth means a new inner balance with no end points. No, your life will never be exactly the same as it was before you were diagnosed with cancer—but it might be more fulfilling.

- Growth means exploring our assumptions about life. Ultimately, exploring our assumptions about life after a brush with a life-threatening illness can make those assumptions richer and more life-affirming.

- Growth means using our potentials. The encounter with cancer reawakens us to the importance of using our potentials—our capacities to mourn our losses openly and without shame, to be interpersonally effective in our relationships with others, and to continue to discover fulfillment in life, living, and loving.

CARPE DIEM
Consider the ways in which you may be growing emotionally and spiritually since your diagnosis.

OUR PRAYER FOR YOU

May the ideas in this book help you embrace and mourn your cancer grief.

May you be surrounded by the love and care of others, and may you let them in whenever they knock.

May you look for beauty even in the ugliest moments.

May you find hope when you need it.

May you nurture your spirit in ways that bring you closer to your self and to God.

May you live with purpose and love each and every day of your remaining life.

May you embrace what your life journey has been teaching you.

May you find untapped stores of compassion within yourself so that you can be kind to yourself as well as help others in need.

May you come to a place where you are ready to unwrap the gifts of cancer.

Blessings to you as you continue to explore your lessons learned, questions asked, and choices made.

We wish you peace and joy!

The Cancer Mourner's
BILL OF RIGHTS

Ten Self-Compassionate Principles

Though you should reach out to others as you journey through cancer grief, you should not feel obligated to accept the unhelpful responses you may receive from some people. You are the one who is experiencing the many losses of cancer, and you have certain "rights" no one can take away from you.

1. **You have the right to your own unique cancer story.**
   Your cancer story is unique. There is only one you. The type and stage of cancer you have are part of your story, yes, but there is so much more to your experience than that. Your age, your gender, your upbringing, your personality, your cancer history, your faith, your relationships—all of these factors and more will shape your unique cancer story. No one else will feel and grieve exactly as you do. So when you turn to others for help, don't allow them to tell you what you should or should not be feeling or thinking.

2. **You have the right to understand cancer as a significant loss.**
   From the moment you are diagnosed with cancer, so many treasured aspects of your life are threatened or lost. Your health, body parts, hair, goals, dreams, intimacy, friends, finances—these and many other things are placed into jeopardy and sometimes lost irretrievably. Of course you grieve deeply. And so you must mourn deeply as well.

3. **You have the right to feel all kinds of emotions.**
   Shock, numbness, fear, guilt, and anger are just a few of the emotions you might experience as part of your grief journey. Others may tell you that some of your feelings are wrong. Don't believe it. Feelings are not right or wrong—they just *are*. Having a feeling inside means you need to express it outside of you.

4. **You have the right to set appropriate limits.**
   The process of cancer diagnosis and treatment is usually extremely tiring and overwhelming. Your feelings of loss will also make you physically and emotionally fatigued. Respect what your body and mind are telling you. Get ample rest each day. Eat balanced and healthy meals. And don't force yourself to do more than you have the energy to do.

5. **You have the right to talk about your cancer grief.**
   Talking about your inner thoughts and feelings will help you cope, survive, and thrive. Seek out others who will allow you to talk as much as you want, as often as you want, about your grief. If at times you don't feel like talking, you also have the right to be silent—as long as you are not closing yourself off to the people who love you.

6. **You have the right to need, ask for, and accept support.**
   In so many ways, cancer is a blitzkrieg. Your body, emotions, mind, social self, and spirit are all under attack. You can't fight this onslaught alone. You need the help of compassionate friends and family members who care about you. They *want* to fight with you, side-by-side. Let them. You also need an excellent care team and maybe a support group of other cancer survivors.

7. **You have the right to ask "Why?"**
   Cancer brings us face-to-face with our most profound questions about life and death. Why do I have to be sick? Why now? Why does anyone die prematurely? Why was I born in the first place? You may or may not find answers to your "Why?" questions. Watch out for the clichéd responses some people may give you. Comments like "It was God's will" or "God wouldn't give you more than you can handle" are not helpful, and you do not have to accept them.

8. **You have the right to embrace (and question) your spirituality.** If faith is a part of your life, express it in ways that seem appropriate to you. Allow yourself to be around people who understand and support your religious or spiritual beliefs. If you feel angry at God or are filled with doubt right now, that's OK too. Find someone to talk to who won't be critical of your spiritual questions.

9. **You have the right to fight if you want to fight…and to give up if you want to give up.** For some people, battling cancer is a prolonged and brutal battle. When is enough enough? Only you can say. You may not be able to control your destiny, but you can control your course of treatment.

10. **You have the right to love and live fully every remaining day of your singular life.** Living and loving fully means being honest, with yourself and with others, about your innermost thoughts and feelings. It means living your truth and connecting with people you care about.

ALSO BY ALAN WOLFELT
AND KIRBY DUVALL

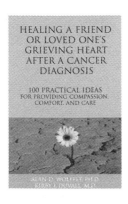

Healing a Friend or Loved One's Grieving Heart After a Cancer Diagnosis

100 Practical Ideas for Providing Compassion, Comfort, and Care

by Alan D. Wolfelt, Ph.D. and Kirby J. Duvall, M.D.

When someone you love is diagnosed with cancer, it's hard to know what to do. What should you say? What shouldn't you say? How can you help? This book will help you understand the normal and natural grief your friend is experiencing. Some of the 100 ideas explain the basic principles of grief and mourning and how they apply to a life-altering, life-threatening, or terminal medical diagnosis. Others offer immediate, here-and-now suggestions of things you can do today to help your friend not only survive but thrive. No matter the type or stage of cancer, the treatment plan, or the prognosis, this compassionate and practical guide will help you be a good companion through the journey that is cancer.

ISBN 978-1-61722-203-0 • 128 pages • softcover • $11.95

Companion
PRESS

All Dr. Wolfelt's publications can be ordered by mail from
Companion Press
3735 Broken Bow Road
Fort Collins, CO 80526
(970) 226-6059
www.centerforloss.com

ALSO BY ALAN WOLFELT

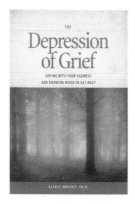

The Depression of Grief

Coping with Your Sadness and Knowing When to Get Help

When someone you love dies, it's normal and necessary to grieve. Grief is the thoughts and feelings you have inside you, and sadness is often the most prominent and painful emotion. In other words, it's normal to be depressed after a loss. This compassionate guide will help you understand your natural depression, express it in ways that will help you heal, and know when you may be experiencing a more severe or clinical depression that would be eased by professional treatment. A section for caregivers that explores the new DSM-5 criteria for Major Depression is also included.

"This enlightening book revealed to me that I am not flawed and it further gave me the strength to go back and do a bit more work so I could truly mourn the loss of my mom and start living life once again." — Kerry Bratton

"This is a much needed resource for both persons who are experiencing grief and professional caregivers who often have a limited understanding of the subtle differences between grief and clinical depression. This book is not only thorough and informative; it is written in a way that is relevant to any person involved in grief and bereavement work." — Jane Castle

ISBN 978-1-61722-193-4 • 128 pages • softcover • $14.95

Companion
PRESS

All Dr. Wolfelt's publications can be ordered by mail from
Companion Press
3735 Broken Bow Road
Fort Collins, CO 80526
(970) 226-6059
www.centerforloss.com

ALSO BY ALAN WOLFELT

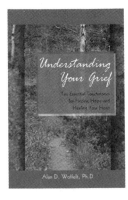

Understanding Your Grief

Ten Essential Touchstones for Finding Hope and Healing Your Heart

One of North America's leading grief educators, Dr. Alan Wolfelt has written many books about healing in grief. This book is his most comprehensive, covering the essential lessons that mourners have taught him in his three decades of working with the bereaved.

In compassionate, down-to-earth language, *Understanding Your Grief* describes ten touchstones—or trail markers—that are essential physical, emotional, cognitive, social, and spiritual signs for mourners to look for on their journey through grief.

The Ten Essential Touchstones:

1. Open to the presence of your loss.
2. Dispel misconceptions about grief.
3. Embrace the uniqueness of your grief.
4. Explore your feelings of loss.
5. Recognize you are not crazy.
6. Understand the six needs of mourning.
7. Nurture yourself.
8. Reach out for help.
9. Seek reconciliation, not resolution.
10. Appreciate your transformation.

Think of your grief as a wilderness—a vast, inhospitable forest. You must journey through this wilderness. To find your way out, you must become acquainted with its terrain and learn to follow the sometimes hard-to-find trail that leads to healing. In the wilderness of your grief, the touchstones are your trail markers. They are the signs that let you know you are on the right path. When you learn to identify and rely on the touchstones, you will find your way to hope and healing.

ISBN 978-1-879651-35-7 • 176 pages • softcover • $14.95

Companion
PRESS

All Dr. Wolfelt's publications can be ordered by mail from
Companion Press
3735 Broken Bow Road
Fort Collins, CO 80526
(970) 226-6059
www.centerforloss.com

ALSO BY ALAN WOLFELT

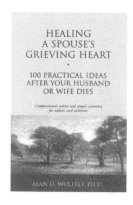

Healing a Spouse's Grieving Heart

100 Practical Ideas After Your Husband or Wife Dies

When your spouse dies, your loss is profound. Not only have you lost the companionship of someone you deeply loved, you have lost your helpmate, your lover, the person you shared your history, and perhaps your financial provider. Learning to cope with your grief and find continued meaning in life will be difficult, but you can and you will if you embrace the principles set down in this practical guide.

This book offers 100 practical, here-and-now suggestions for helping widows and widowers mourn well so they can go on to live well and love well again. Whether your spouse died recently or long ago, you will find comfort and healing in this compassionate book.

ISBN 978-1-879651-37-1 • 128 pages • softcover • $11.95

Companion
PRESS

All Dr. Wolfelt's publications can be ordered by mail from
Companion Press
3735 Broken Bow Road
Fort Collins, CO 80526
(970) 226-6059
www.centerforloss.com

ALSO BY ALAN WOLFELT

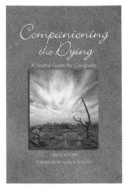

Companioning the Dying
A Soulful Guide for Caregivers

by Greg Yoder, Foreword by Alan D. Wolfelt

Based on the assumption that all dying experiences belong not to the caregivers but to those who are dying—and that there is no such thing as a "good death" or a "bad death" —*Companioning the Dying* helps readers bring a respectful, nonjudgmental presence to the dying while liberating them from self-imposed or popular expectations to say or do the right thing.

Written with candor and wit by hospice counselor Greg Yoder, who has companioned several hundred dying people and their families, *Companioning the Dying* exudes a compassion and a clarity that can only come from intimate work with the dying. The book teaches through real-life stories that will resonate with both experienced and clinical professionals as well as laypeople in the throes of caring for a dying loved one.

ISBN 978-1-61722-149-1 • 148 pages • softcover • $19.95

Companion
PRESS

All Dr. Wolfelt's publications can be ordered by mail from
Companion Press
3735 Broken Bow Road
Fort Collins, CO 80526
(970) 226-6059
www.centerforloss.com

TRAINING AND SPEAKING
ENGAGEMENTS

To contact Dr. Wolfelt about speaking engagements or training opportunities at his Center for Loss and Life Transition, email him at DrWolfelt@centerforloss.com.